UNDERSTANDING

MELANOMA

What You Need to Know

5th Edition

by

Perry Robins, MD
Maritza Perez, MD

Published by

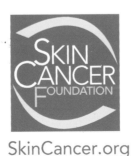

SkinCancer.org

Understanding Melanoma, What You Need to Know, 5th Edition

by

Perry Robins, MD

Maritza Perez, MD

Copyright © 1996, 2005, 2006, 2010, 2015 by The Skin Cancer Foundation

ISBN-13: 978-1-329-30798-8

Published by The Skin Cancer Foundation

149 Madison Avenue, Suite 901, New York, NY 10016

SkinCancer.org

info@skincancer.org

THE SKIN CANCER FOUNDATION

The Skin Cancer Foundation is the only organization devoted entirely to combating the most common cancer in the world today. A non-profit foundation, it carries out educational programs on sun protection, early warning signs of skin cancer, and the need for prompt, effective treatment. The Foundation's melanoma campaign is dedicated to raising awareness of this disease. Such programs have won the Excellence in Education Award and 16 Gold Triangle Awards for community service from the American Academy of Dermatology, as well as the Advertising Club of New York's Andy Award of Excellence and the Telly Award honoring outstanding film and video productions and commercials.

THE AUTHORS

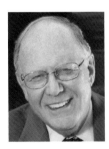

Perry Robins, MD, is the Founder and President of The Skin Cancer Foundation. He is Professor Emeritus of Dermatology and former Chief of the Mohs Micrographic Surgery Unit at New York University Medical Center. Dr. Robins has been honored for distinguished service by the four leading dermatologic societies and is chairman of skin cancer conferences in the US and around the world. He is the founder-president of the International Society for Dermatologic Surgery, founder/former president of the American College of Mohs Micrographic Surgery, and former president of the American Society of Dermatologic Surgery. He has published extensively in major medical journals, authored 5 books, and is the founder of the the the *Journal of Dermatologic Surgery* and the *Journal of Drugs in Dermatology*. Dr. Robins has been named an honorary member of 11 international dermatology societies.

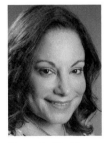

Maritza I. Perez, MD, Founder and Director of Advanced Dermaesthetics in New Canaan, CT, is Director of Cosmetic Dermatology at Mt. Sinai/Roosevelt Hospital Center, Associate Director of Procedural Dermatology at Beth Israel Medical Center, and Associate Professor of Clinical Dermatology at Mount Sinai Icahn School of Medicine in New York City. She is a recipient of the Dermatology Foundation Award and Fellowship and The Skin Cancer Foundation's Joseph G. Gaumont Fellowship in Dermatologic Surgery with Dr. Perry Robins at New York University Medical Center in New York City. Dr. Perez is also a Senior Vice President of The Skin Cancer Foundation.

ACKNOWLEDGMENTS

As physicians, we have seen the need for a handbook that offers information and hope to melanoma patients, their families, friends, and others deeply concerned with the most serious of all skin cancers.

So much has taken place in the field since **Understanding Melanoma,** first published in 1996, was revised and updated for a fourth edition in 2010 that a fifth edition is needed to provide readers with the most recent information.

We wish to recognize the many people who have helped with this and the previous editions of **Understanding Melanoma**. Above all, we appreciate the effort and commitment of the staff of The Skin Cancer Foundation. Mary Stine and Mitzi Moulds, present and former Executive Directors, have provided strong leadership and expert guidance, and Mark Teich has served as executive editor of the last two editions.

Jean Bolognia, MD, Alfred W. Kopf, MD, Ruth Oratz, MD, and Allan C. Halpern, MD, helped us by serving as Medical Reviewers and offering valuable insights. Derek Jones, MD, receives our thanks for all his help.

Physicians have reported that this book has been extremely useful, and melanoma patients have told us how helpful and reassuring it was to them. We would like to thank the many people who have supported and encouraged us.

DEDICATION

To my children, Elizabeth and Lawrence, and all patients with melanoma—may they have long, healthy, happy lives. **P.R**

To my parents, my husband, my daughters, and my colleagues—you have all been instrumental in advancing my career and helping me to complete this book successfully. **M.P.**

TABLE OF CONTENTS

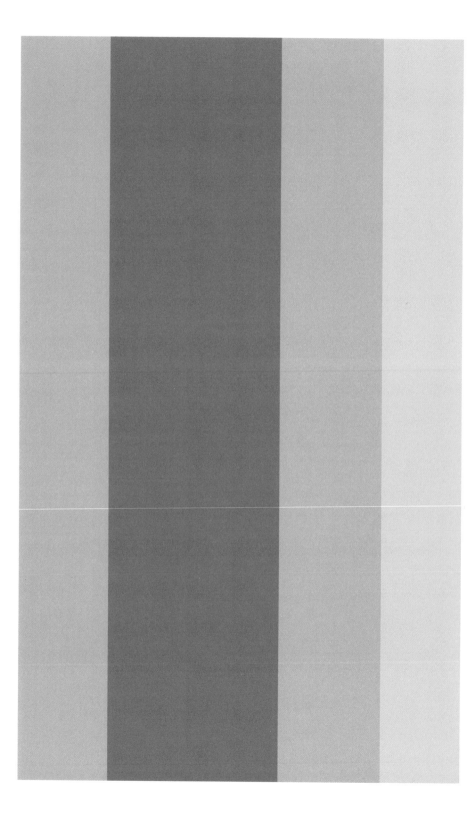

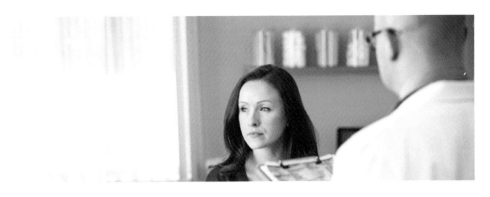

Introduction

AFTER THE DIAGNOSIS

"You have a melanoma."

Anyone who has heard a physician make that statement will remember the shock and anxiety that followed.

Often the person had no idea that anything was wrong and came for a routine examination. In other cases, the physician visit was scheduled out of no more than a mild concern about an odd-looking mole or discolored spot. The discovery that there is a serious problem produces a feeling of bewilderment, a sense of knowing far too little about the disease.

"What is a melanoma?"

That is the first question most often asked.

And then, in hopes that the physician's report might be wrong —

"Are you sure there's no mistake?"

The third question is the one that came to mind the instant the word "melanoma" was spoken.

"Is it fatal? Am I going to die?"

You will find the answers to the questions asked by melanoma patients, their family members, and every other person concerned with the disease in **Understanding Melanoma**: *What You Need to Know*. That is why we felt it was so important to write this handbook. Especially with recent advances in early detection and treatment, the facts are probably more positive than you think they are, the future more hopeful.

As you read the chapters on diagnosis and treatment, you will see that a diagnosis of melanoma does not have to be the end. It is not as bad as most people believe. There is an excellent chance for a long and healthy life after the diagnosis.

The vast majority of people with melanoma are cured. In fact, if the melanoma is discovered and treated while it is thin and limited to the uppermost layer of the skin, the long-term survival rate is 98 percent.

When these thin melanomas are included in calculating the average overall five-year survival rate, it stands at more than 90 percent. Consider that only 80 year ago fewer than 13 percent of people with melanoma lived this long, and you can see how far medicine has advanced and how the odds have changed in favor of the patient.

Melanoma is not a minor illness. It is much more dangerous than the most common forms of skin cancer — basal cell and squamous cell carcinoma. If it is overlooked and, therefore, left untreated until it has spread through the body, it is life-threatening. Nowadays that happens less often than in the past, and even when it does, new medical advances in treatments can improve the outlook.

REMEMBER:

THERE IS LIFE

AFTER THE DIAGNOSIS.

CHAPTER 1
WHAT IS MELANOMA?

Melanoma is the most serious form of skin cancer. That is the simplest answer to the question.

Patients, their families, and other concerned people want to know more. To reach a more complete understanding, it is necessary to learn how the cells in the body become malignant.

The Origin of Melanoma

Melanoma is a malignant tumor that originates in melanocytes, the cells which produce melanin, the pigment that colors our skin, hair, and eyes and is heavily concentrated in most moles. The majority of melanomas, therefore, are black or brown. However, melanomas occasionally stop producing pigment. When that happens, the melanomas may no longer be dark, but are skin-colored, pink, red, or purple.

Which Are More Serious?

The physician will tell you whether the melanoma is early or more advanced by describing it as either *in situ* or invasive. *In situ* is Latin and means "in one site" or "localized." Melanomas *in situ* occupy only the uppermost part of the epidermis, the top layers of the skin. They have not penetrated deeper.

Invasive melanomas are more serious, as they have penetrated more deeply into the skin and may have spread cells from the original tumor through the body.

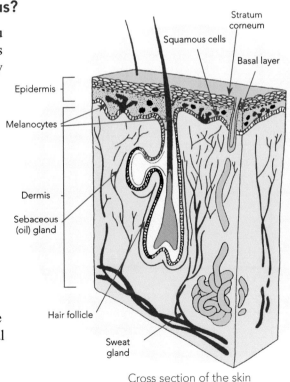

Cross section of the skin

THE FOUR BASIC TYPES

Melanomas fall into four basic categories. Three of them begin *in situ* and sometimes become invasive; the fourth is invasive from the start. It is helpful to recognize the names and be able to define the characteristics of each type.

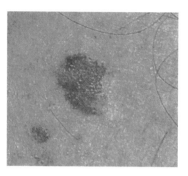

Superficial spreading melanoma, the most common type, arising from an atypical (odd-looking) mole.

Superficial spreading melanoma is by far the most common type, accounting for about 70 percent of all cases. As its name suggests, this melanoma grows along the top layer of the skin for a fairly long time before penetrating more deeply.

The first sign of it is the appearance of a flat or slightly raised discolored patch that has irregular borders and is somewhat asymmetrical in form. The color is rather dark, and you may see areas of tan, brown, black, red, blue, or white. Sometimes an older mole will change in these ways, or a new one will arise. A melanoma can be found almost anywhere on the body, but is most likely to occur on the trunk in men, the legs in women, and the upper back in both. Trunk melanomas, however, have been increasing in incidence in women, possibly due to increased indoor and outdoor tanning. Most melanomas found in the young are of the superficial spreading type.

Lentigo maligna is similar to the superficial spreading type, but it usually remains

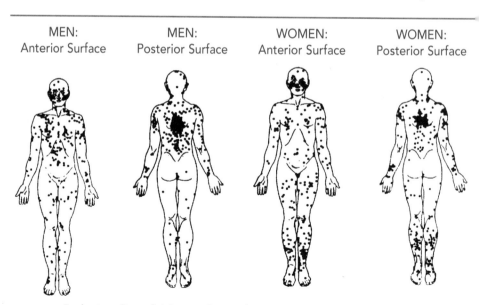

Body sites. Superficial spreading melanoma appears almost anywhere, but most often on the trunk in men, legs in women, and upper back in both.

Lentigo maligna arises on chronically sun-exposed skin.

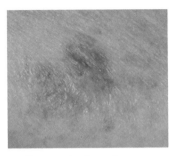

Desmoplastic melanoma

close to the skin surface for quite a while, and most often appears as a flat or mildly elevated, mottled tan, brown, or dark brown discoloration.

This type of *in situ* melanoma is found most often in the elderly, arising on chronically sun-exposed, damaged skin on the face, ears, arms, and upper trunk. Lentigo maligna is the most common form of melanoma in Hawaii.

When this cancer becomes invasive, it is referred to as lentigo maligna melanoma (about six percent of all melanomas).

Desmoplastic melanomas are a variant of the disease most often associated with lentigo maligna melanoma and the invasive vertical growth phase of a lesion, though the most common early clinical evidence of it is a preinvasive, radial (horizontal) growth phase along the surface of the epidermis, during which a macular pigmentation (dark, flat spot) resembling a freckle, solar lentigo, or lentigo maligna appears. These melanomas involve pervasive deposits of collagen or desmin (dense protein filaments found in muscle cells) around the tumor and are regarded as variant patterns of spindle cell melanoma, consisting primarily of spindle cells (elongated cells tapered at both ends) rather than the more common epithelioid, or round, cells.

Clinically, these unusually fibrous, often non-pigmented tumors may initially appear to be something other than melanomas, which may account for why they were once considered rare; they are now being reported more often because of the general rise in melanoma incidence and because pathologists and clinicians have become more familiar with their features. They can still present a diagnostic challenge to the clinician, and special stains have been developed to help distinguish them from other growths. They are most often found on sun-exposed areas of the head and neck, especially in elderly individuals, though rare cases have been discovered in patients as young as 13 years old. Partly related to their tendency to involve the nerves, invasive melanomas with desmoplastic features are often locally aggressive, with a poor prognosis, but like other melanomas, they carry a better prognosis when diagnosed early and properly treated.

The third type of melanoma, **acral lentiginous melanoma** (ALM, about 5 percent of melanomas), also spreads superficially before penetrating more deeply. It is quite different from the others, though, as it usually appears as a black or brown discoloration under the nails or on the soles of the feet or palms of the hands, areas with minimal sun exposure. Believed to be caused by other, unknown factors, it is sometimes found in dark-skinned people, and can often advance more quickly than superficial spreading melanoma and lentigo maligna. It is the most common melanoma in African-Americans and Asians, accounting for 15 to 35 percent of all cases, and the least common among Caucasians.

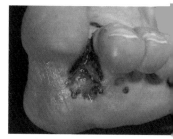

Acral lentiginous melanoma (or ALM) on the sole of a brown-skinned patient's foot

Nail bed (subungual) melanoma is a type of ALM that typically shows up on the nails of the thumb or big toe in one of two ways: as a dark brown to black streak that extends from the cuticle to the tip of the nail (called *longitudinal melanonychia*), or as a so-called "colorless" tumor (known as *amelanotic melanoma)* that may actually be red, pink, purple, or normal skin tone. Unfortunately, nail melanomas are often mistaken for less serious conditions until they are at an advanced stage. They can be mistaken for bruises, injuries, ingrown toenails, calluses, warts, fungi, or sores, and thus ignored. Consequently, diagnosis is often delayed, leading to poorer outcomes.

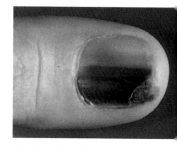

Nail bed melanomas may show up as a dark brown to black streak called "longitudinal melanonychia" that extends from the cuticle to the tip of the nail.

Unlike the other three types, **nodular melanoma** (10 to 15 percent of melanoma cases) is usually invasive at the time it is first diagnosed. The malignancy is recognized when it becomes a bump. The color is most often black, but occasionally blue, gray, white, brown, tan, red, or skin tone.

The most frequent locations are the trunk, legs, and arms, mainly of elderly people, as well as the scalp in men. This is the most aggressive of the melanomas.

Many patients feel they do not know what questions to present to the physician. The information given in this handbook will help you to ask the right questions and get the right answers.

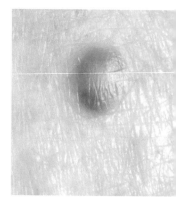

Nodular melanoma with a blue-black hue.

CHAPTER 2

MAKING THE DIAGNOSIS

"How did you make the diagnosis?
Are you sure there's no mistake?"

Anyone who hears the diagnosis of melanoma naturally hopes an error has been made, and it is true that a mole may look like a melanoma and turn out to be a harmless skin growth. For that very reason, a physician will not give a diagnosis until the pathology testing has been completed. Modern diagnostic laboratory techniques have been perfected to the point where they are virtually always correct in showing whether a mole is cancerous or benign (noncancerous).

Biopsy: the Basis for Diagnosis

Every diagnosis begins with a thorough examination of the skin growth or pigmented lesion under a bright light. If the physician sees anything to arouse suspicion, a tissue biopsy will then usually be performed. This is the most accurate diagnostic test.

The goal is to remove the tumor totally, although this may not be possible when it is large or located in a hard-to-reach location, such as the nailbed. At the start of the procedure, a local anesthetic is usually administered by a fine needle. Then the tissue is surgically removed with a scalpel. If the lesion is small, the physician may cut through the full thickness of the skin down to the underlying fat, and take some of the surrounding skin as well; in such cases, the tumor might be removed in its entirety. If the tumor is more extensive, only a small sample of the involved area will be surgically excised. The wound may then be closed by suturing (stitching).

There will often be a scar at the site of the biopsy, but in most cases, this is not cosmetically disfiguring.

Laboratory Studies

The biopsy sample (specimen) is sent to a pathology laboratory where it is prepared and stained for examination under the microscope. The result of this finding as to whether the lesion is benign or malignant is then provided to the physician. If it is malignant, the cancer is classified according to type and thickness. Most melanomas are recognized in this way.

In some cases, the diagnosis is not clear-cut, and it may be wise to get a second opinion from a pathologist who specializes in melanoma. Certain moles mimic the appearance of melanoma, and certain melanomas mimic the appearance of other cancers or even of benign moles. In such cases, microscopic examination of the tissue (histologic examination) may not be conclusive. To establish the diagnosis, a number of highly sophisticated stains have been developed. These stains make use of antibodies, which are formed as an immune response to the antigen or molecule on the surface of the tumor cells. An antibody attaches itself to only one type of antigen. Therefore, a number of different antibodies are tested to see whether reactions to any of the antigens expressed by the tumor cells take place.

In rare instances, the diagnosis may still not be definitive after these tests. Researchers today are refining new **"microarray technologies"** to enhance diagnostic certainty in the future. These techniques, which began with the first studies of the human genome in the 1990s, allow scientists to screen large numbers of genes, examining DNA with great sensitivity not just on the organic but on the molecular level. Researchers are attempting to harness these technologies to study the patterns of gene activity in different lesions. Damage to our DNA (by exposure to ultraviolet light or other causes) can result in significant changes (mutations) in genes that lead to cancers, and the microarray techniques may allow scientists to measure and catalog these changes. By detecting the varying expression and function of these different mutated genes, the scientists hope to distinguish melanomas from benign moles or other cancers.

Dermoscopy Aids in Decision-Making

You may also hear about the use of dermoscopy as a diagnostic tool. (Dermoscopy is occasionally referred to by other names, epiluminescence microscopy or dermatoscopy.) This procedure, which is painless, makes use of a handheld instrument called the **dermoscope** or **dermatoscope.** It can provide the physician with an enlarged, more detailed view of the lesion providing more information than is obtained with the naked eye, and is useful in distinguishing benign pigmented lesions from melanoma or other malignant pigmented lesions.

Until recently, all dermoscopes used *non-polarized* light that required direct contact with a liquid or gel (for example, oil or water) between the dermoscope and the skin. This solution was spread on the pigmented lesion and the area around it to make the skin more translucent. One end of the dermoscope's eyepiece was immersed in the liquid and pressed against the skin, and the physician looked at the lesion through a magnifying lens. This technique was called non-polarized dermoscopy (NPD).

Modern dermoscopes use *cross-polarized* light, which does not require the liquid interface or in some cases even direct contact. Polarized *contact* dermoscopy (PCD) uses polarized light with direct contact while polarized *non-contact* dermoscopy (PNCD) works without direct contact. NPD, PCD, and PNCD each have something different to offer in achieving a precise diagnosis.

The features that can be identified with a dermoscope include a "network" resembling a fisherman's net made up of pigment, brown globules, black dots, and color variations. A variety of algorithms (precise step-by-step instructions for analysis) are now used to study these features, first to determine if a lesion is pigmented or not (melanocytic or non-melanocytic), and then to help determine whether it is malignant or not.

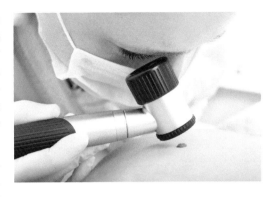

Dermoscopic examination assists the dermatologist in deciding whether a biopsy is needed by helping to indicate the likelihood of melanoma. Many patients, therefore, may be spared the need for undergoing biopsies. For example, one of the newer dermoscopy algorithms is the **Beauty and the Beast** technique: the dermoscopic pattern of the lesion is compared against nine established, typical benign patterns, and if it strays from any of these patterns, a biopsy should be considered.

Nail (subungual) lesions, among others, are good candidates for dermoscopy. Although subungual melanomas often start as a dark stripe under the nail, not all of these streaks represent melanoma. Dermoscopy can help differentiate melanomas from benign pigmented streaks. Signs of subungual melanoma that show up under dermoscopy include brown or black background discoloration, pigmentation of the cuticle known as a micro-Hutchinson's sign, irregularly spaced pigmented bands on the nail, and irregular thickness, color, or ridge patterns.

New Imaging Methods Hold Promise

Many new *automated* imaging systems are now under investigation in hopes of improving upon clinical and dermoscopic precision in melanoma diagnosis, and several have been approved by the FDA in the past few years. Some of these include:

Image Analysis and Computer-Assisted Diagnosis

Numerous computer programs can objectively document the clinical and dermoscopic features of digitized pigmented lesion images. Most rely on sophisticated programs to determine the boundary separating the lesion from normal skin, and then, once the computer identifies the lesion, the program utilizes features programmed in as characteristic of melanoma, such as multiple colors, uneven texture, asymmetry, and border irregularity. Most systems analyze the images, providing "computer–assisted diagnosis" approaching or exceeding the sensitivity and specificity achieved by expert dermoscopists.

Confocal Scanning Laser Microscopy (CSLM)

This technique makes use of a low-power visible or near-infrared laser, a scanning microscope, and a computer with software to enhance digitized pictures. It allows real-time *(in vivo)* examination of the epidermis and papillary dermis (the topmost part of the dermis, immediately below the epidermis) at a high resolution. It can provide instant high-resolution images of the cell structures and sometimes even subcellular structures of a lesion before the decision is made to do a biopsy. The technique is becoming an accepted method for distinguishing between melanomas and benign lesions. Multiple CSLM units are available and FDA-approved, including new versions with miniaturized, more user-friendly handheld confocal scanners, such as the VivaScope 3000.

Multi-spectral Imaging and Automated Diagnosis (spectrophotometric analysis): Knowing that light of different wavelengths penetrates skin to different depths led investigators to evaluate pigmented lesions under wavelengths from infrared to near ultraviolet. Two systems—the SIMSYS-MoleMate™ SIAscope™ (Spectrophotometric Intracutaneous Analysis system) and MelaFind[R]—employ such "multi-spectral" sequences of dermoscopic images for computer analysis. The SIAscope™ requires physician interpretation, while MelaFind[R] provides a diagnosis in a completely automated system. Both often enable physicians to see the constituents of skin without cutting it open; they formulate or negate a melanoma diagnosis prior to biopsy. Both techniques were FDA-approved in 2011.

The SIMSYS-MoleMate™ SIAscope™, a handheld device, uses both visible and infrared light to examine skin components such as blood, melanin, dermal melanin, and collagen to a depth of 2-2.5 mm below the skin surface in a pain-free, noninvasive manner, providing gross living pathological data on suspicious skin lesions. Siascopy can eliminate the need for more laborious clinical examination and laboratory analysis procedures. Using sophisticated mathematical models and software programs, SIAscopy generates bitmap images called SIAscans, which can either be displayed on PCs, viewed separately, or overlaid, to demonstrate how skin features relate to one another. This allows physicians to know the exact size of a lesion and make more precise incisions.

MelaFind[R] is a noninvasive and objective computer vision system intended to aid in early detection of melanoma. Before a final decision to biopsy has been made, MelaFind[R] acquires and displays multi-spectral (10 distinct wavelengths from blue to near infrared) digital images of pigmented skin lesions, such as atypical moles, and employs automated image analysis and statistical pattern recognition to evaluate the degree of three-dimensional disorganization in the tumor. Highly disorganized tumors should be biopsied to rule out or diagnose melanoma.

It is important to remember that all of these techniques and systems are just helpful, complementary tools to aid in diagnosis; none of them are substitutes for an experienced physician.

CHAPTER 3

HOW SERIOUS IS IT?

Establishing the diagnosis of melanoma is just the beginning. The next step is to classify the disease by degree of severity.

The biopsy report gives the physician a sound basis for evaluation. The stage of the melanoma is then determined by means of further physical examination and additional laboratory studies. This information is of vital importance to the patient.

Four Stages

In giving a melanoma diagnosis, the physician will tell the patient the stage number assigned to the melanoma — from Stage I through Stage IV, with Stage I the earliest and Stage IV the most advanced. Early melanomas are localized, and advanced melanomas have spread, or to use the technical term, *metastasized*. Each stage has been defined according to certain specifications, which will be described in detail in this chapter.

The information may seem complicated at first glance, because the medical terms are not in common use. Do not get discouraged. There is a logical progression from one stage to the next, which is not difficult to grasp. Once you know the characteristics of each, the diagnosis will be much easier to understand.

GUIDE TO STAGING

New Melanoma Staging System – By means of an unprecedented cooperative effort among cancer centers around the world, the classification system recommended by the American Joint Commission on Cancer (AJCC) was updated in 2010. Approval was based on clinical experience with close to 40,000 melanoma patients. New findings about melanoma were incorporated to allow for the most accurate diagnosis and prognosis (a forecast of how the disease is likely to progress).

Formerly, very thin tumors were classified according to **Clark's level of invasion,** the number of layers of skin penetrated by the tumor. In the newest staging system, Clark's level has far less importance.

The most important factors in the new staging system are the thickness of the tumor, known as **Breslow's thickness** (also called **Breslow's depth**), the appearance of microscopic **ulceration** (meaning that the epidermis on top of a major portion of the melanoma is not intact), and **mitotic rate**, the speed of cell division (how fast the cancer cells are growing). Clark's level will enter into serious consideration only in the rare instances when mitotic rate cannot be determined.

To be exact, Breslow's thickness measures in millimeters (1 mm equals 0.04 inch) the distance between the upper layer of the epidermis and the deepest point of tumor penetration. The thinner the melanoma, the better the chance of a cure. Therefore, Breslow's thickness is considered one of the most significant factors in predicting the progression of the disease.

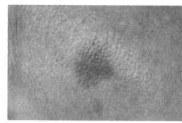

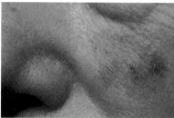

• *In situ* (noninvasive) melanoma remains confined to the epidermis.

• Thin tumors are less than 1.0 millimeter (mm.) in Breslow's depth.

• Intermediate tumors are 1.0-4.0 mm.

• Thick melanomas are greater than 4.00 mm.

Two examples of thin melanomas.

The presence of microscopic ulceration upgrades a tumor's seriousness and can move it into a later stage. Therefore, the physician may consider using a more aggressive treatment than would otherwise be selected.

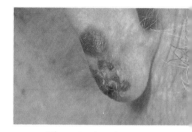

Mitotic rate was introduced into the staging system based on recent evidence that it is also an independent factor predicting prognosis. The

Ulcerated melanoma.

presence of at least one mitosis (cancer cell division) per millimeter squared (mm^2) can upgrade a thin melanoma to a later stage at higher risk for metastasis.

Early Melanomas (Clinical Stages 0 and I)

Early melanomas (Stages 0 and I) are localized; Stage 0 tumors are *in situ*, meaning they are noninvasive and have not penetrated below the surface of the skin, while Stage I tumors have invaded the skin but are small; they may or may not be ulcerated, and may or may not be growing at a slow mitotic rate. They are not known to have spread anywhere else in the body, though Stage Ib tumors may be at higher risk of spreading to the lymph nodes.

STAGE II TUMORS, though localized, are larger (generally over 1 mm. thick) and may be ulcerated or have a mitotic rate of greater than than $1/mm.^2$ They are at heightened risk of spreading to nearby lymph nodes.

There are several subdivisions within these tumor stages:

T categories (for Tumor)

- **Stage Tis.** The tumor is in situ and remains non-invasive in the epidermis.
- **Stage T1a.** The tumor is less than or equal to 1.0 mm in Breslow's thickness, without ulceration and with a mitotic rate of less than $1/mm^2$.
- **Stage T1b.** The tumor is less than or equal 1.0 mm thick. It is ulcerated and/or the mitotic rate is equal to or greater than $1/mm^2$.
- **Stage T2a.** The tumor is 1.01-2.0 mm thick without ulceration.
- **Stage T2b.** The tumor is 1.01-2.0 mm thick with ulceration.
- **Stage T3a.** The melanoma is 2.01-4.0 mm thick without ulceration.
- **Stage T3b.** The melanoma is 2.01-4.0 mm thick with ulceration.
- **Stage T4a.** The tumor is thicker than 4.0 mm without ulceration.
- **Stage T4b.** The tumor is thicker than 4.0 mm with ulceration.

Later Stages

ADVANCED MELANOMAS (Stages III and IV) have metastasized to other parts of the body – Stage III beyond the tumor as far as to nearby lymph nodes, and Stage IV to distant parts of the body, potentially including vital organs.

Stage III. By the time a melanoma advances to Stage III or beyond, an important change has occurred. The Breslow's thickness is by then irrelevant and is no longer included in staging, but the presence of microscopic ulceration continues to be used, as it has an important effect on the progression of the disease. At this point, the tumor has metastasized beyond the original tumor site, either to the nearby lymph nodes or to the skin between the primary tumor and the nearby lymph nodes. (The latter are called in-transit or satellite metastases.) All tissues are bathed in lymph—a colorless, watery fluid consisting mainly of white blood cells—which drains into lymphatic vessels and lymph nodes throughout the body, potentially carrying cancer cells to distant organs.

Whether or not a tumor has metastasized to the nearby lymph nodes can be determined by examining a biopsy of a specific node in the local lymphatic basin; appropriately called the "sentinel node," this is the first node into which the lymph fluid from the tumor drains, often the first node in the basin. However, sometimes lymph from the tumor drains into more than one node, meaning there are multiple sentinel nodes. A sentinel node biopsy (SLNB) is now generally done when a tumor is more than 1 mm in thickness, or when a thinner melanoma of 0.76 mm or more shows evidence of ulceration and/or a high mitotic rate. As SLNB is not considered necessary in all cases, you may wish to discuss the matter with your physician. You will read more about the sentinel node in Chapter 4.

In-transit or satellite metastases, included in Stage III, have spread to skin or underlying (subcutaneous) tissue for a distance of more than 2 centimeters (1 cm equals 0.4 inch) from the primary tumor, but not to the regional lymph nodes.

In addition, the new staging system includes metastases so tiny they can be seen only through the microscope (micrometastases). Just how advanced the tumor is into Stage III (the "N" category, for "nodes") depends on factors such as whether the metastases are in-transit or have reached the nodes, the number of metastatic nodes, the number of cancer cells found in them, and whether or not they are micrometastases or can be felt (palpated) or seen with the naked eye.

Stage IV. The melanoma has metastasized to lymph nodes distant from the primary tumor or to internal organs, most often the lung, followed in descending order of frequency by the liver, brain, bone, and gastrointestinal tract. The two main factors in determining how advanced the melanoma is into Stage IV (the M category, for "metastases") are the site of the distant metastases (non-visceral, lung, or any other visceral metastatic sites) and elevated serum lactate dehydrogenase (LDH) level. LDH is an enzyme released into the blood when cells are damaged or destroyed.

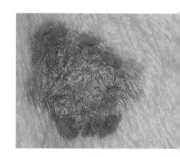

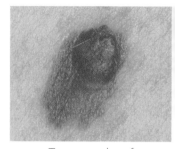

Two examples of intermediate melanomas

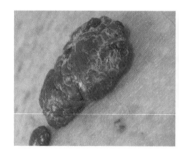

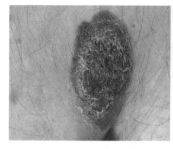

Two examples of thick melanomas

Understanding Melanoma

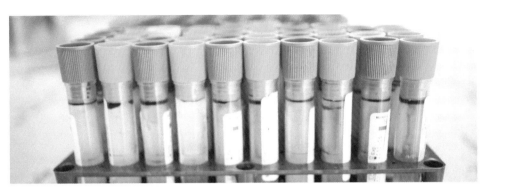

CHAPTER 4

TREATMENT ADVANCES

What does the future hold? Anyone who has had a diagnosis of melanoma is worried. It is a natural reaction, and some people believe their future is bleak. Fortunately, that is not usually true. When it comes to early-stage disease, the future could hardly be brighter. Most people with thin, localized melanomas are cured by appropriate surgery.

Therefore, you can see that the sooner the cancer is caught and treated, the better the results. Early detection remains the best weapon in fighting melanoma.

However, even for those with more advanced disease, there is good news, as the cure rate keeps rising. The treatments are varied and many; new discoveries are being made every day to improve the chances of those with metastatic disease, and in the past few years, the FDA has approved several revolutionary therapies that are significantly extending lives, with some patients essentially cured. There is a very real possibility that in the not-distant future, advanced melanoma could change from a deadly to a chronic, survivable disease.

Surgical Techniques Improve

Excision of Primary Melanoma

The first step in melanoma treatment is removal of the tumor, and the standard method is surgical excision (cutting it out). Surgery has made great advances in the past decade, and much less tissue is removed than was customary in the past. Patients do just as well after the lesser surgery, which is easier to tolerate and produces a smaller scar.

The surgical excision is also called resection, and the borders of the entire area excised are known as the margins.

Outpatient /Office Surgery

In most cases, the surgery for thin melanomas can be done in the doctor's office or as an outpatient procedure under local anesthesia. Stitches (sutures) remain in place for one to two weeks, and most patients are advised to avoid heavy exercise during this time. Scars are usually small and improve over time.

Discolorations and areas that are depressed or raised following the surgery can be concealed with cosmetics specially formulated to provide camouflage. If the melanoma is larger and requires more extensive surgery, a better cosmetic appearance can be obtained with flaps made from skin that is near the tumor, or with grafts of skin taken from another part of the body. For grafting, the skin is removed from areas that are normally or easily covered with clothing.

There is now a trend towards performing sentinel node biopsy and tumor removal surgery at the same time, provided the tumor is 1 mm or more in thickness or is ulcerated.

Setting the Margins

In the new approach to surgery, much less of the normal skin around the tumor is removed. The margins, therefore, are much narrower than ever before. This spares significant amounts of tissue and reduces the need for postoperative cosmetic reconstructive surgery. Most US surgeons today follow the guidelines recommended by the National Institutes of Health and the American Academy of Dermatology Task Force on Cutaneous Melanoma.

- When there is an *in situ* (noninvasive) melanoma, the surgeon excises 0.5-1 centimeter of the normal skin surrounding the tumor and takes off the skin layers down to the fat. To kill any residual unseen cancerous cells, some doctors may consider the use of radiation therapy or imiquimod cream, a topical therapy that stimulates the immune system to produce interferon, a chemical that attacks cancerous and precancerous cells.

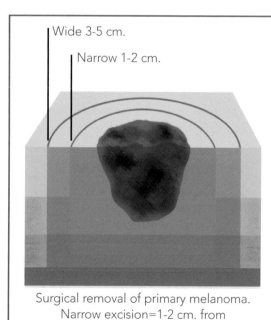

Wide 3-5 cm.

Narrow 1-2 cm.

Surgical removal of primary melanoma. Narrow excision=1-2 cm. from tumor border. Wide excision=3-5 cm.

- In removing a melanoma that is 1 mm or less in Breslow's thickness, the margins of surrounding skin are extended to 1 cm and the excision goes through all skin layers and down to the fascia (the layer of tissue covering the muscles).

- If the melanoma is 1.01 to 2 mm thick, a margin of 1-2 cm is taken.

- If the melanoma is 2.01 to 4 mm thick, a margin of 2 cm is taken.

- If the melanoma is greater than 4 mm thick, a margin of 2 cm is still taken.

These margins all fall within the range of what is called "narrow" excision. When you consider that until recently, margins of 3 to 5 cm (wide excision) were standard, even for comparatively thin tumors, you can see how dramatically surgery has changed for the better. Physicians now know that even when melanomas have reached a thickness of 4 mm or more, increasing the margins beyond 2 cm does not increase survival.

Mohs Micrographic Surgery

In recent years, Mohs Micrographic Surgery, which many physicians consider the most effective technique for removing basal cell and squamous cell carcinomas (the two most common skin cancers), is being increasingly used as an alternative to standard excision for certain melanomas. In this technique, one thin layer of tissue is removed at a time, and as each layer is removed, its margins are studied under the microscope for the presence of cancer cells. If the margins are cancer-free, the surgery is ended. If not, more tissue is removed, and this procedure is repeated until the margins of the final tissue examined are clear of cancer.

Mohs surgery thus can eliminate the guesswork in the removal of skin cancers and pinpoint the cancer's location when it is invisible to the naked eye. Mohs surgery differs from other techniques since the microscopic examination of all excised tissues during the surgery eliminates the need to "estimate" how far out or deep the roots of the skin cancer go. This allows the Mohs surgeon to remove all of the cancer cells while sparing as much normal tissue as possible.

In the past, Mohs was rarely chosen for melanoma surgery for fear that some microscopic melanoma cells might be missed and end up metastasizing. In recent years, however, efforts to improve and refine the Mohs surgeon's ability to identify melanoma cells have resulted in the development of special stains that highlight these cells. These stains are known as immunocytochemistry or immunohistochemistry (IHC) stains and use substances that preferentially stick to pigment cells (melanocytes), where melanoma occurs, making them much easier to see with the microscope. For example, staining excised frozen tissue sections with *melanoma antigen recognized by T cells (MART-1)* effectively labels/locates the melanocytes, helping to home in on melanomas. The MART-1-stained sections are processed and evaluated for the presence of tumor in the margins; certain signs such as nests of atypical melanocytes show that the margins are

The Steps Involved in Mohs Surgery

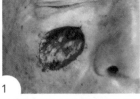

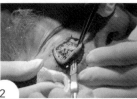

1

1. *Original tumor site is presented*

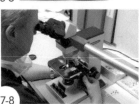

2

2. *Tissue is removed*

3. *Tissue is inked for orientation*

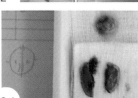

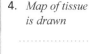

3-4

4. *Map of tissue is drawn*

5. *Tissue is sectioned and placed on a glass slide*

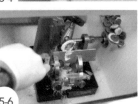

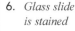

5-6

6. *Glass slide is stained*

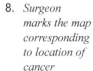

7. *Surgeon examines slide and identifies residual cancer*

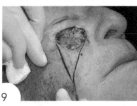

7-8

8. *Surgeon marks the map corresponding to location of cancer*

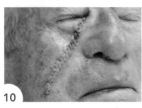

9

9. *Surgeon returns to bedside with map to precisely excise remaining cancer*

10

10. *Process is repeated until no cancer remains; wound is closed*

positive for melanoma and that further surgery must be done. If none of these signs are present, the surgery is concluded.

Thanks to such advances, more surgeons are now using the Mohs procedure with certain melanomas.

Lymph Node Involvement

Once the melanoma has progressed beyond Stage II, it has spread beyond the original site. It is most likely to have reached the lymph nodes that are closest to the tumor. You have read about the lymphatic system in the previous chapter.

Palpable nodes. To find out whether melanoma cells have escaped the primary tumor, the physician starts by feeling the nearby lymph nodes. If the melanoma is on the arm, the nearest nodes are in the armpit; if on the leg, they are in the groin. For a melanoma on the head, the closest lymph nodes are usually on the neck on the same side. For a tumor on the trunk, the nodes in either the armpit or the groin could be involved.

When there is an enlargement or lump in a lymph node, it is described

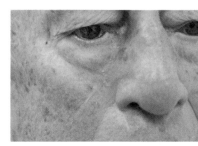

Two years after the surgery

as "palpable," meaning that the physician can feel it on physical examination. A palpable lymph node is almost always surgically removed today. It is then sent to the pathology laboratory to be tested microscopically for the presence of malignant cells. If any are found, the rest of the nodes in that basin will also be removed, and treatments that stimulate the immune system (immunotherapies) and/or chemotherapy will be recommended.

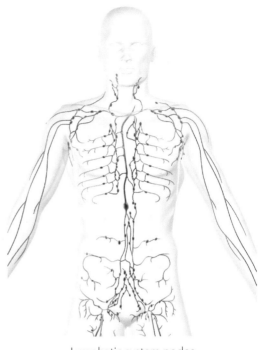
Lymphatic system nodes

Non-palpable nodes. The lymph nodes are not always palpable even when melanoma cells have spread beyond the original tumor. In the past, there was much debate about when to excise and examine the local lymph nodes. Depending on how early the tumor was, some believed in a wait and see policy; others believed in removing all the nodes (*radical node dissection*) in the region of the tumor on the chance there were hidden cancer cells; this was called elective lymph node dissection, or ELND.

Lymphoscintigraphy (Lymphatic Mapping) and Sentinel Node Biopsy

Today, there are specific guidelines for when to investigate the regional lymph nodes. Two techniques refined over the past two decades, *lymphoscintigraphy* and *sentinel node biopsy* (*SLNB*, described in chapter 3), have solved the problem of whether or not to perform radical lymph node dissection in the absence of clinically palpable nodes.

Generally, when patients have melanomas under 1 mm in thickness, with no ulceration and a mitotic rate of less than $1/mm^2$, nodal dissection is deemed unnecessary. For melanomas that have reached 1 mm in thickness, and/or have ulceration or a mitotic rate of $1/mm^2$ or greater, lymphoscintigraphy and SLNB are undertaken to determine whether all the nodes in the regional lymph node basin should be removed.

Lymphoscintigraphy is a technique for mapping the lymphatic pathway to track whether melanoma cells have metastasized from the primary melanoma tumor to the local lymph nodes. A small amount of a harmless radioactive substance is injected at the site of the melanoma to trace the flow of lymph fluid draining from it to the nodes. Then, with the help of a scanner, the drainage pattern of the lymph fluid is determined. Sulfur colloid has been the chief radioactive tracer drug used but in 2013, a new tracer called Lymphoseek (technetium Tc99m tilmanocept) became the first new radioactive tracer for lymph node mapping to be FDA-approved in more than 30 years, after studies proved it to be especially effective at locating the lymph nodes.

Most often, a second lymphatic mapping technique is also used to increase certainty: a blue dye (isosulfan blue) is injected into the skin around the tumor, and the dye passes into the lymph fluid, tracing its path. The blue color is picked up first by the node closest to the tumor, which is referred to as the sentinel node. Sometimes there are one or more other sentinel nodes as well, which should also show up in the dye and radioactive tracer tests.

Armed with the findings from this lymphatic mapping, the surgeon can at first remove only the sentinel nodes. Once a specific area (basin) of lymph drainage has been pinpointed by the dye or tracer, the sentinel node(s) can be removed surgically and tested in the pathology laboratory, the premise being that if any melanoma cells reach the local nodal basin, they will hit the sentinel node(s) first. If no cancer cells are found in the sentinel nodes, no further surgery is performed. If cancer cells are present in the sentinel nodes, the rest of the nodes in this lymphatic basin will also usually be removed and examined. Once melanoma cells are confirmed in the lymph nodes, the patient is reclassified as Stage III, and additional (adjuvant) treatment with the immunotherapy interferon alfa-2b and/or other treatments will usually be instituted after the radical lymph node dissection in an attempt to keep the cancer from recurring.

In 2013, Lymphoseek became the first new radioactive tracer for lymph node mapping to be FDA-approved in more than 30 years.

Though sentinel node biopsy is now considered the standard of care for patients whose melanomas are considered at high risk of spreading to the lymph nodes, some debate about the technique remains. There is no doubt that it avoids more radical surgery in patients whose sentinel nodes prove negative for melanoma, and it is universally acknowledged to be an important technique for determining prognosis and staging, and thus for planning treatment. However, it has not been definitively proven that the technique (or *any* lymph node surgery) extends patients' overall survival.

Early in 2014, a long-awaited study (the Multicenter Selective Lymphadenectomy Trial-1, or MSLT-1) did not prove extended overall survival or melanoma-specific survival, but did show that SLNB is associated with improved *recurrence-*

Understanding Melanoma

free survival (the length of time before recurrence). In another recent study of melanoma patients with primary lesions over 1 mm in thickness, published in *Annals of Surgery*, van der Ploeg, et al found that over all, patients who were merely observed after their primary melanoma tumors were removed by wide local excision had comparable melanoma-specific survival to those who underwent SLNB after the wide local excision. However, those patients whose melanomas specifically ranged *from 1.0 to 4.0 mm in thickness* had significantly improved disease-free survival and regional recurrence-free survival, as well as improved *distant metastasis-free* survival, after SLNB, compared to observation only.

It is hoped that MSLT-2, an ongoing follow-up trial of MSLT-1, will help resolve the remaining questions.

Research is now also exploring special biochemical techniques that can identify any melanoma cells that do not show up in the course of routine microscopic examination and sentinel node biopsy.

In Europe and Australia, ultrasound is also frequently used before SLNB and during follow-up for detection of lymph node metastases. A new ultrasound avenue is guided fine-needle aspiration cytology, performed before SLNB. This minimally invasive technique may decrease the need for some SLNBs; patients whose sentinel nodes test positive in ultrasound can proceed straight to radical dissection. A large multicenter, multicountry validation study may help determine the future use of ultrasound for detection of lymph node metastases.

Local Vs. Distant Spread

Once the disease has advanced to Stage IV, melanoma cells have traveled through the body via the bloodstream or lymph vessels, going far from the original tumor site. They may have reached distant lymph nodes or invaded the internal organs. This can be in addition to or instead of in-transit metastases or local spread to the regional lymph nodes. In local forms of the disease, the metastases can reach skin or subcutaneous tissue more than 2 cm from the primary tumor, but not beyond the regional lymph nodes.

When distant metastases are suspected, they can be traced by scans of the chest, head, abdomen, and pelvis with a CT (computed tomography) scan in which special x-ray equipment and a computer program show a cross section of body tissues or organs; an MRI (magnetic resonance imaging) scan that uses a magnet instead of x-ray to create a map of the patient's body and brain; and by PET (positron emission tomography), an established but evolving radiographic technique. For PET scanning, radioactive sugar, the basic carbohydrate utilized by the body for energy, is injected intravenously into the patient. This sugar may be taken up rapidly by any melanoma cells that are present.

Additional (Adjuvant) Treatment

When cancer cells spread to the lymph nodes and beyond (Stages III and IV), the melanoma is considered advanced, and a variety of treatment options are now available. The patient can ask the physician to explain the possibilities and ground for selection of one adjuvant over the other. These additional treatments include radiation, chemotherapy, immunotherapy (using mass-produced synthetic versions of natural immune system chemicals, or inhibiting proteins that block the immune system), and the more recently developed *targeted* therapy, as well as combinations of these treatments. These techniques do not cure the majority of advanced cancers. However, they often delay the cancer's advance for months or even years and offer tremendous hope for patients who previously had little. Some advanced melanoma patients have now survived for several years, and researchers believe that in the near future, this will be the rule rather than the exception.

Chemotherapy

A number of drugs that are active in fighting cancer cells are being used to treat melanoma, either one at a time or in combinations. Currently, Dacarbazine (DTIC) given by injection, is the only chemotherapy approved by the Food and Drug Administration (FDA) for Stage IV melanoma. DTIC may be combined with carmustin (BCNU) and tamoxifen, or with cisplatin and vinblastine. Temozolomide (Temodar®), an oral drug closely resembling DTIC, is FDA-approved for brain cancers but also used off-label for melanomas that have spread to the brain or nervous system. Other drugs may be substituted for DTIC or added to it.

To date, the response of melanomas to chemotherapy has been limited, and other treatments are usually tried first, but some promising chemotherapies are being tested. One new type of chemotherapy that has received considerable attention in the media is a class of drugs known as *anti-angiogenic*. This medical term means that they prevent new blood vessels from forming. This is important because they can cut off the blood supply that would otherwise nourish the cancer cells and enable them to grow. These drugs are still in early experimental stages for melanoma (though they are FDA-approved for some other cancers), and a good deal of research into improving and combining them with other therapies is going on. However, early results for some anti-angiogenic agents, including bevacizumab (Avastin), thalidomide, endostatin, and sorafenib have been disappointing, and have not shown any survival advantage.

> Early results with some anti-angiogenic agents have been disappointing, and have not shown a survival advantage.

Isolated Limb Perfusion Method: This palliative treatment, which relieves symptoms, is sometimes used when melanoma metastases have reached an arm or leg. "Isolation" means that the chemotherapy is "perfused" (shunted directly) to the blood flowing through the affected limb, but to no other part of the body, to limit toxic effects. The drug melphalan is the chemotherapy most frequently used, often combined with other agents.

Immunotherapy (Also Known as Biologic Therapy or Biotherapy)

This is one of the most exciting and changing fields in medicine, based on drugs that act on the body's immune system. To date, the most successful treatments for advanced melanoma have been immunotherapies, with some recently FDA-approved treatments offering many patients substantially increased lifespans verging on cures.

For Stage II high-risk patients and Stage III patients: The first immunotherapy to be FDA-approved (in 1995) was injectable *interferon (IFN) alfa-2b,* a mass-produced version of an immune chemical occurring naturally in the body. High-risk melanomas are tumors that have a high chance of recurring (such as those that are ulcerated or over 4 mm thick) or have spread to the nearby lymph nodes. At first, IFN alfa-2b appeared to increase overall 5-year survival. After further study, it proved to give patients a longer period without relapse, extending their disease-free interval to an average of 9 months, but did not lengthen overall survival. It has significant flu-like side effects.

In 2011, the FDA approved an improved version of IFN alpha-2b called *pegylated interferon alfa-2b* or *peginterferon alfa-2b* (also known as Sylatron™), to treat Stage III melanoma patients. The drug, injected subcutaneously like its predecessor, was approved following a trial in which melanoma patients taking Sylatron™ remained relapse-free an average of nine months longer than patients not taking the drug (34.8 months vs. 25.5 months). The difference between this new drug and its predecessor was the addition

> **About 10-16 percent of Stage IV patients on high-dose IL-2 respond to it, and about 60 percent of those have significantly extended lives.**

of the chemical polyethylene glycol to the interferon, through the process known as pegylation; this enhanced the half-life of the interferon compared to its original form—meaning that the effects of the treatment lasted longer, enabling patients to remain relapse-free longer. However, to date there has been no significant difference in length of overall survival.

For Stage IV patients: The first FDA-approved immunotherapy for Stage IV patients was injectable high-dose **interleukin-2, or IL-2,** also called **Proleukin**, a mass-produced version of a *lymphokine* (an immune chemical naturally produced by the white blood cells in small quantities) that enters melanoma cells and attacks them. Approved in the late 1990s, high-dose IL-2 is associated with very significant side effects, but has been found to increase disease-free and overall survival in some patients. About 10-16 percent of carefully selected patients on IL-2 regimens respond to the drug, with six percent having *complete* responses (remissions), and about 60 percent of the complete responders have significantly extended lives.

Tumor-infiltrating lymphocytes (TILs) also play an exciting part in some new immunotherapies for advanced melanoma. Of special note is a technique from the National Cancer Institute called *adoptive cell transfer (ACT)*, still in clinical testing, which involves harvesting TILs from the patient's blood, then isolating from them the cells expressing T cell receptors that can recognize melanoma-specific antigens; in other words, the most aggressive melanoma-killing lymphocytes are identified and isolated. These are then grown in large numbers in the lab and re-injected into the patient in the hope that they will massively attack the patient's melanoma cells. High doses of IL-2 may be added to make these tumor-fighting cells mature and multiply, and certain drugs are used to eliminate immune factors that might inhibit the tumor-fighting cells; this is called *lympodepletion*. In clinical trials with metastatic melanoma patients who had not responded to previous treatment, the patients' response rates have been far higher than those seen with chemotherapy. In the latest trials, total-body irradiation was added to enhance lymphodepletion. ACT with TILs as part of a lymphodepleting regimen has been shown in clinical trials to cause objective clinical responses in approximately 40-72 percent of metastatic melanoma patients, with up to 40 percent of those patients experiencing complete responses (remissions) lasting up to 7 years ongoing. According to Dr. Steven A. Rosenberg at the National Cancer Institute, a pioneer in this technique, ACT is a potentially curative therapy. Ongoing trials to simplify the regimens may allow a broader range of patients to be treated.

The most successful form of melanoma immunotherapy to date is "**checkpoint blockade therapy,**" which now boasts three recently FDA-approved drugs that are significantly extending lives for many metastatic melanoma patients.

The first successful checkpoint blockade therapy was **ipilimumab (Yervoy®)**, approved in 2011 for patients with advanced melanoma. Ipilimumab is a monoclonal antibody (a purified class of antibodies cloned and mass-produced in the lab from one specific type of cell or cell line) that blocks CTLA-4 (cytotoxic T-lymphocyte-associated protein 4), which is a kind of natural "brake" in the immune system that can inhibit activation of T cells, thereby preventing them from destroying the tumor. Ipilimumab is considered an "anti-CTLA-4 therapy": It inhibits CTLA-4 so that more T cells can be produced to fight the melanoma. Ipilimumab has yielded dramatic, sustained responses akin to cures in certain patients. In a study of 1,861 patients treated with ipilimumab, about 22 percent lived three years or longer, and 84 percent of those survivors were alive after 5 years and 10 years. One recent report, in fact, suggested that 20 percent of patients who received ipilimumab are alive after 10 years. In contrast, only about 4-6 percent of patients were ever found to achieve long-term survival with interleukin-2, and no overall survival advantage was ever demonstrated with chemotherapy.

In 2014, two additional immune checkpoint-blockading drugs, pembrolizumab (Keytruda®) and nivolumab (Opdivo®), were FDA-approved. Both inhibit another molecule called programmed death-1, or PD-1, that, like CTLA-4, prevents T-cells from attacking the melanoma. PD-1 can directly interact with tumor cells by binding to a molecule called programmed death ligand-1 (PD-L1), and cancer cells may use PD-L1 to hide from attack by T-cells, but these drugs can release the T-cells to fight the cancer.

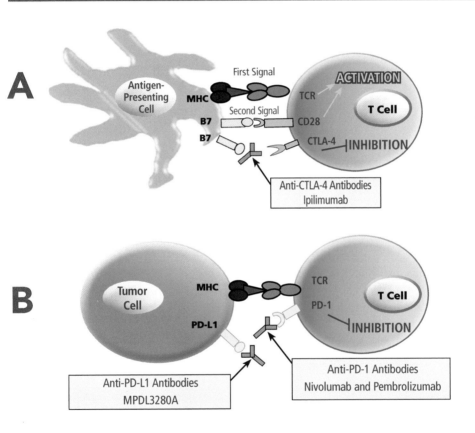

MHC= major histocompatibility complex, TCR=T-cell receptor

CTLA-4 and PD-1

A. In lymphatic tissue, antigen-presenting cells (APC) activate naïve T-cells via the T-cell receptor (TCR) and stimulatory receptor CD28. This leads to expression of CTLA-4 on the T-cell surface, which binds to B7, leading to T-cell inactivation. Ipilimumab binds to CTLA-4 and reverses this inactivation.

B. In peripheral tissue, tumor cells upregulate PD-1 ligands, which bind to PD-1 on activated T-cells, leading to T-cell inhibition or death. Monoclonal antibodies that bind to either PD-1 or PD-L1 interfere with this, allowing antitumor T-cells to survive and kill the tumor cells.

Both pembrolizumab and nivolumab are approved for use in patients:

- whose melanoma has metastasized or cannot be removed by surgery;
- and who have had disease progression after treatment with ipilimumab;
- and who, if they have an abnormal BRAF gene, have had disease progression following treatment with a targeted BRAF inhibitor (vemurafenib or dabrafenib).

Other PD-1 inhibitors for advanced melanoma are in the wings, and a related inhibitor dubbed *MPDL3280A* blocks PD-L1, the ligand that binds PD-1 to T cells and deactivates them. Thus far, PD-1/PD-L1 blockades have resulted in even higher response rates, progression-free survival and overall survival rates, as well as a more favorable side effect profile than that seen with ipilimumab. Many researchers have begun asserting that they should become front-line therapies, rather than be reserved for patients who have already been treated with ipilimumab or a BRAF inhibitor. Several randomized trials comparing ipilimumab with anti-PD-1 therapy are ongoing, and to date, the studies show that the anti-PD-1 therapies are even more effective than ipilimumab.

In October 2015, the FDA gave accelerated approval to *combination* nivolumab-ipilimumab for patients with metastatic or inoperable melanoma, based on the CheckMate -069 trial, which found that the combination therapy demonstrated a 60 percent reduction in disease progression compared to ipilimumab alone. Approved for patients who do not have the mutated BRAF gene (see "Targeted Therapies" on p. 27), this is the first combination immunotherapy ever approved for patients with cancer. The trial showed median progression-free survival of 8.9 months with the combination regimen, vs. 4.7 months for ipilimumab alone, with *17 percent* of all patients on the combination therapy going into remission.

Ipilimumab, pembrolizumab, and nivolumab have yielded dramatic sustained responses akin to cures.

In a new development that could be a huge boon to patients, the checkpoint blockade therapies could soon start to be used earlier *before* Stage IV, when they may save even more lives. Recently the FDA accepted an application for ipilimumab to be used for Stage III patients at high risk of recurrence, after their tumor and local lymph nodes are removed. Here, it would be used as an "adjuvant" therapy – a supplementary treatment to prevent recurrences and metastasis beyond the lymph nodes. Acceptance of the application was based on results from a Phase III trial showing a 25 percent improvement in recurrence-free survival in Stage III patients treated with ipilimumab versus placebo. This trial is the first to show that the checkpoint blockade drugs may be given earlier in the course of disease, when they can do more good and potentially cure more patients.

The FDA is scheduled to make a decision on ipilimumab as a Stage III adjuvant therapy by October 28 of 2015.

Yet another new direction in immunotherapy is injectable **oncolytic viruses**—viruses injected directly into tumors to preferentially infect the cancer cells while leaving healthy cells intact. The most advanced of these intralesional therapies in clinical trials is *talimogene laherparepvec*, or *T-VEC*. When T-VEC, a modified herpes virus that can't infect the patient, is injected into a melanoma tumor, it selectively infects the tumor, rupturing its cell walls. T-VEC has been encoded with the human gene for a molecule called *granulocyte-macrophage stimulating factor* (GM-CSF), which can help boost the immune system to fight cancer throughout the body. The hope is that as the tumor disintegrates, it will release infectious virus particles carrying the GM-CSF, thereby stimulating inflammatory signals that broadly activate the immune system so that T-cells attack other, non-inoculated tumors. Thus, both the virus and the immune system itself attack the tumor. Both Phase II and Phase III studies have had striking results. The Phase III study, presented at the 2014 American Society of Clinical Oncology annual meeting, produced a 16 percent response rate vs. 2 percent in the untreated control patients, and nearly 40 percent of the responses were complete responses (remissions).

Based on the results so far, two FDA panels have voted 22-1 recommending approval of T-VEC for metastatic melanoma patients.

In a recent Phase Ib trial of previously untreated stage IIIB-IV melanoma, T-VEC was combined with ipilimumab in the hopes that the latter would augment the tumor-killing response throughout the body, and that T-VEC might speed up patients' response to ipilimumab.

Targeted Therapies

Targeted therapies, among the most revolutionary treatments for advanced melanoma, use drugs or other substances to identify and attack specific types of cancer cells, or to block the action of certain genes, enzymes, proteins or other molecules that promote the growth and spread of cancer cells. This allows the cancerous cells to be treated without killing healthy cells.

The past few years have brought several notable successes in targeted melanoma therapy. The first was vemurafenib (Zelboraf®), FDA-approved in 2011, which inhibits the defective BRAF gene. BRAF, part of the mitogen-activated protein kinase (MAPK) pathway that when defective can promote melanoma growth, produces a protein that normally regulates skin cells, causing them to multiply only when growth is needed. However, a specific mutated version of BRAF called V600E (found in about half of all melanoma patients)—and in smaller subsets of patients, the related mutant gene versions V600K and V600D—produces an abnormal version of the protein that stays switched on. This leads to out-of-control growth, i.e., cancer. In patients with the defective BRAF gene, vemurafenib can bind to the defective protein and deactivate it. Studies have shown that it produces strik ing and rapid antitumor activity in patients with BRAF V600E- and V600K-mutate melanoma, leading to both a progression-free and overall survival (OS) advantage i vemurafenib patients compared to standard chemotherapy (median OS of 13. months for vemurafenib patients vs. 9.7 months for chemotherapy patients).

While this is a significant increase in survival, and while some patients go muc longer before recurrence, most patients eventually develop resistance to the trea ment, and the melanoma starts to grow and advance again.

In the hope of solving the problem, in 2013 two other targeted treatments wer approved by the FDA, one also directed at BRAF and one at a related molecu called MEK, downstream of BRAF in the MAPK cascade: the BRAF inhibitc dabrafenib (Taflinar®) and the MEK inhibitor trametinib (Mekinist™). All three c these targeted therapies can be used only in patients who have the defective BRA gene. The idea is that even when the BRAF inhibitors vemurafenib and dabrafeni meet with resistance in inhibiting melanoma, trametinib will inhibit its progres sion at MEK further down the MAPK cascade, at least delaying the melanoma' advance.

In 2014, the FDA also approved the use of dabrafenib and trametinib *in combina tion* for patients with inoperable or metastatic melanoma with a BRAF V600 or V600K mutation. The hope is that different drugs and drug combinations wi increase tumor shrinkage and extend the length of time before the melanoma be comes resistant and starts growing again.

Results from the latest studies show that a remarkable *51 percent* of BRAF mutated metastatic melanoma patients on combination dabrafenib-trametinib ar still alive at two years, with median survival of 25.6 months, vs. 45 percent o patients on dabrafenib alone and 38 percent of patients on vemurafenib alon (median survival 18 months).

In addition, a Phase III study of a new BRAF/MEK inhibitor combination the BRAF inhibitor vemurafenib plus an experimental MEK inhibitor calle *cobimetinib* – found that patients with advanced melanoma lived significantly lon ger (almost four months longer) on average than patients on vemurafenib alone Based on these results, cobimetinib has now been submitted to the FDA, and coul be approved sometime in 2015. All these findings have driven researchers to an ticipate a time in the near future when the combination BRAF-MEK inhibitors wi become standard treatment for BRAF-mutant melanoma, phasing out the single drug therapies.

In another direction for targeted therapy, researchers are targeting *C-KIT,* th receptor for an enzyme called tyrosine kinase, which has been associated wit melanoma. Genetic aberrations or mutations in KIT have been frequently foun in certain gastrointestinal tumors and leukemias, which have responded well t targeted treatment, and some limited types of melanoma also frequently have KI mutations, so it has been hypothesized that these melanomas will similarly respond to targeted therapies. Some patients, especially those with acral lentiginous melanoma and mucosal melanoma, have initially responded well to drugs targeting *C-KIT*, including *imatinib* (**Gleevec**) and *nilotinib* (**Tasigna**), but significant clinical improvements from these drugs as single therapies have been minimal. They are continuing to be tested in different dosage regimens and combined with other therapies.

Combining Targeted Therapy and Immunotherapy

Both targeted drugs and immunotherapy are now important treatment options, though the best ways to use them are not yet clear. By killing melanoma cells, BRAF and MEK inhibitors may increase activation of immune cells to attack any remaining melanoma cells, so it may be particularly attractive to combine them with ipilimumab, nivolumab, pembrolizumab, or other checkpoint-blockade immunotherapies. However, initial attempts to combine a BRAF inhibitor (vemurafenib) with immune-checkpoint blockade therapy (ipilimumab) were deemed unsafe, so this combination should not currently be used in standard practice. Clinical trials are now evaluating different combinations of these drugs used in different ways—for example, using them in sequence rather than concurrently. The goal will be to determine which combinations and methods are most suitable to shrink melanoma most effectively, maintain the best possible quality of life for patients and extend patients' lives as long as possible. Many other novel approaches are also on the horizon, currently either in active laboratory study or clinical trials; the hope is to turn metastatic melanoma from a deadly disease into a manageable chronic condition.

Gene therapy: A gene is the basic unit of genetic material. It is the code or "blueprint" by which our body's proteins are made. Alterations in these codes can result in uncontrolled cell growth as in cancer. However, selected genes can be altered so as to correct genetic defects or enhance the cancer-fighting potential of cells. The hope is that making changes in genes will lead to successes in treating a wide range of illnesses.

One form of gene therapy is based on creating alterations in the white blood cells or in the tumor-infiltrating lymphocytes [TILs] so that they will attack the melanoma. This is achieved by removing these cells from the patient, growing them outside the body, and treating them so as to increase their number. The next step is the addition of genetic material that produces one of many growth factors which make the lymphocytes more aggressive as cancer-fighters. These more aggressive lymphocytes are returned to the patient's body in an effort to stimulate the immune system to kill the melanoma and its metastases. (See the discussion of TILs and *adoptive cell transfer* on page 24.)

In a sense, the targeted therapies we discussed before are also forms of genetic therapy, because they target proteins like BRAF and c-KIT produced by genes that have become defective, turning into oncogenes (cancer-producing genes). These defective proteins get stuck in the "on" position, causing uncontrolled cell growth and treatments like vemurafenib, dabrafenib, and trametinib bind up or block those proteins, turning off the uncontrolled growth and in effect correcting the defective gene, at least for a certain period of time.

A possibility for the more distant future might be attempting to alter inherited mutant versions of genes such as *CDKN2A* (*p16*) and the so-called "redhaired" variants of the melanocortin 1 receptor gene (MC1R), which are passed from generation to generation in certain families or ethnic groups, leaving family members at highly increased risk of developing melanoma. However, such treatments are in very early stages of research.

One focus of current research is the identification of genes for specific melanoma antigens. These are molecules found on the cell wall, and they stimulate the production of antibodies, which are a part of the body's immune defense system. As explained in chapter 2, an antibody attaches itself to only one type of antigen. By injecting the gene for the melanoma antigens, the hope is to increase their number and produce a broad attack by the patient's immune system. But again, such treatments are in very early stages of research.

Possibilities

Many patients, especially those with advanced disease, are participating in clinical trials in order to receive new treatments while they are still experimental and not generally available. Such is the case with drugs such as imatinib and nilotinib, targeting c-KIT, and the PD-L1 inhibitor MPDL3280A. At present, patients can obtain such treatments only in clinical trials.

Remember, just a few short years ago, ipilimumab, nivolumab, pembrolizumab, and the BRAF-based targeted therapies were available only in clinical trial as well, and now they are all approved, widely available, and significantly extending lives. More effective treatment possibilities exist than ever before, and more are coming, giving realistic new hope to people with advanced melanoma.

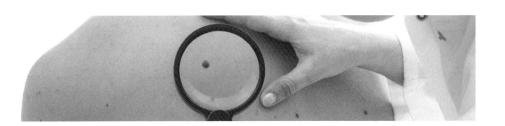

CHAPTER 5

EARLY WARNING SYSTEMS

When a melanoma is detected at an early stage and treated, a cure is all but certain. Many, if not most, melanomas can be spotted as soon as they arise — if you know what to look for and check for those signs.

FIVE WARNING SIGNS: THE ABCDES

There are five basic warning signs of a melanoma called the ABCDEs:

A stands for **Asymmetry.** If you were to draw a line through the middle of the melanoma, the two sides would not match. This is in contrast to a common, benign mole, which is round and symmetrical.

B stands for **Border.** Melanomas are frequently irregular in shape, with scalloped or notched edges. In contrast, a common harmless mole has smooth, even borders.

C stands for **Color.** Melanomas display a variety of shades of brown or black, as well as some unusual shades — mixed red, white, and blue. In contrast, common moles generally are a rather uniform shade of brown.

D stands for **Diameter.** The melanoma is usually larger than 1/4 inch (6 millimeters) in diameter (not to be confused with Breslow's thickness), the size of a pencil eraser. There are some exceptions, however, and a melanoma may be smaller when first detected.

E stands for **Evolving** or changing. This is the newest addition to the signs now recognized as differentiating ordinary moles from early melanomas, and it is the first sign you should consider. If you have a mole that changes in any way, or if a new mole appears, see your doctor.

The Ugly Duckling Sign

While the ABCDE rule helps detect many melanomas, some melanomas do not exhibit the ABCDE features. Recently, several melanoma specialists developed a new method of sight detection for skin lesions that could prove to be melanoma. This method is based on the concept that these melanomas look different—they are "ugly ducklings"—compared to surrounding moles. The premise is that the patient's "normal" moles resemble each other, like siblings, while the potential melanoma is an "outlier," a lesion that, at a given moment in time, *looks* or *feels* different than the patient's other moles, or that over time, ***changes differently*** than the patient's other moles. The ugly duckling methodology may be especially useful in the detection of nodular melanoma, a dangerous type of melanoma, which notoriously lacks the classic ABCDE signs.

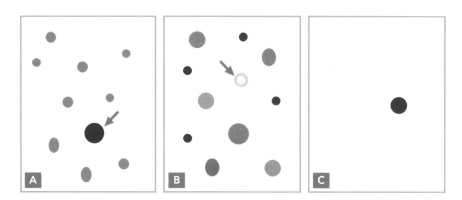

These three different scenarios depict ugly duckling moles that should prompt suspicion. Squares A, B, and C each represent a body area such as the back.

- In A, there is a dominant mole pattern with slight variation in size. The ugly duckling is clearly darker and larger than all other moles.

- In B, there are two main patterns, one of larger moles and the other of smaller, darker moles. The ugly duckling is small but lacks pigmentation.

- In C, there is only one lesion on the back. If this lesion is changing, symptomatic, or deemed atypical, see a doctor and have this ugly duckling examined.

Thus, during skin self-examination and professional examination, patients and physicians should be looking for lesions that manifest the ABCDE's, AND for lesions that look different compared to surrounding moles. An approach combining the ABCDEs and the Ugly Duckling technique should improve the chances of early detection of all types of melanoma.

The CUBED Guide for Nail Melanomas

The warning signs of nail (subungual) melanoma, a form of the sometimes virulent acral lentiginous melanoma, may also differ from the classic ABCDE signs. Due to frequent misdiagnosis, a panel of medical experts has developed the *CUBED* guide for early recognition of nail melanoma, as well as all foot melanomas. CUBED is an acronym based on a checklist of conditions that indicate the need for a specialist's opinion:

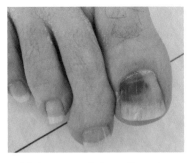

Melanomas of the nail can be mistaken for recent injury.

- **C** = Colored lesions

- **U** = Uncertain diagnosis

- **B** = Bleeding under the nail and the appearance of beefy red tissue

- **E** = Enlargement or deterioration of the lesion or the wound area despite treatment, and

- **D** = Delay in healing beyond two months.

The EFG Rule for Nodular Melanomas

Like nail melanomas, nodular melanomas may not be recognizable using the ABCDEs, since they are often symmetrical, have regular borders, and do not have variegated colors. Experts have thus adopted an additional or alternative acronym called the EFG rule that has proven useful: **E**levated, **F**irm on palpation, and **G**rowing progressively for over a month.

The Blue-Black rule: This is also especially valuable with nodular melanomas. It involves pattern recognition like the ugly duckling technique, drawing attention to any darkly pigmented lesion containing some dark blue and black color that doesn't resemble other surrounding lesions. Again, it is more sensitive for nodular melanoma than the ABCDEs, but combining them achieves even greater accuracy.

HOW MIGHT A MOLE EVOLVE?

Watch for the evolution or change in:

- **Size.** The mole suddenly or continuously gets larger.

- **Color.** A wide variety of colors or color combinations appears. Color might spread from the edge into the surrounding tissue.

- **Elevation.** A mole that was flat or slightly elevated increases in height.

- **Surrounding skin.** Becomes red or develops other color changes.

- **Surface.** A smooth mole develops scaliness, erosion, oozing. Crusting, ulceration, or bleeding may appear late in the course of the disease.

- **Sensation.** Itching is the most common early symptom, and there may also be feelings of tenderness or pain. Nonetheless, remember that skin cancers are usually painless in their early stages.

If any of these changes occurs, or if a new mole appears after age 25, it should be checked by a professional. Look for a physician who specializes in skin cancer and is trained to recognize a melanoma at its earliest stage. Make an appointment without delay. Prompt action is your best protection.

These are the most common differences between normal moles and melanomas, but any suspicious-looking mole should be examined:

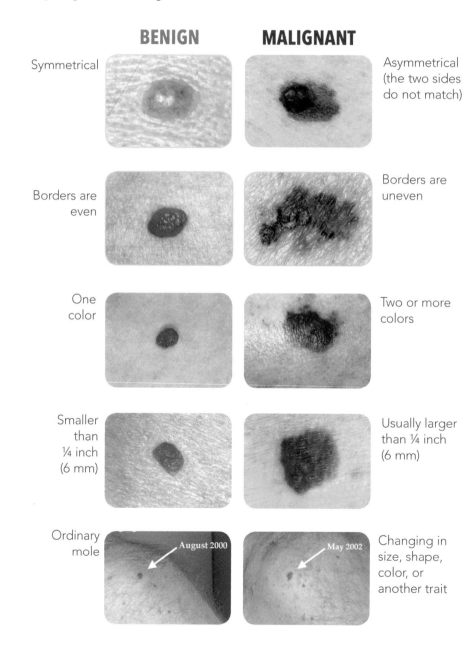

BENIGN	MALIGNANT
Symmetrical	Asymmetrical (the two sides do not match)
Borders are even	Borders are uneven
One color	Two or more colors
Smaller than ¼ inch (6 mm)	Usually larger than ¼ inch (6 mm)
Ordinary mole	Changing in size, shape, color, or another trait

August 2000

May 2002

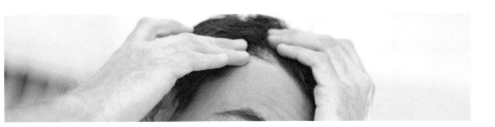

CHAPTER 6

SELF-EXAMINATION COULD SAVE YOUR LIFE

"Skin cancer: If you can spot it, you can stop it." This is the memorable slogan of The Skin Cancer Foundation's lifesaving self-examination campaign.

You are now familiar with the changes in moles that point to possible malignancy, and early warning signs of melanoma such as the ABCDEs and the Ugly Duckling. The next step is to apply this knowledge by visually examining your skin. That is the best way to spot melanoma, as well as the more common nonmelanoma skin cancers, primarily basal cell carcinomas and squamous cell carcinomas.

Examination of the Skin

The standard time scheme for performing self-examination of the skin is once a month. Add to this an annual examination by a dermatologist or other physician experienced in skin care. A more frequent schedule is recommended for those who are at increased risk of melanoma. Your doctor will tell you how often this should be. (You will find risk factors for melanoma described in the next four chapters.)

Because some cancers may arise on parts of the body that are normally covered, all clothes should be removed for a skin examination. The chances of finding a melanoma are six times greater if you completely undress than if you just take off part of your clothing.

Self-Examination Tips

You do not need any elaborate equipment to perform a visual self-examination of your skin. Everything you need is probably in your home already:

- A bright, overhead direct light from a ceiling fixture or floor lamp
- A full-length mirror
- A hand mirror
- Two chairs or stools (or one of each)
- A blow-dryer.

Here are eight simple steps to follow in performing total-body skin self-examination:

1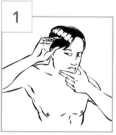
Examine your face, especially the nose, lips, mouth, and ears—front and back. Use one or both mirrors to get a clear view.

5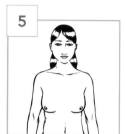
Next, focus on the neck, chest, and torso. Women should lift breasts to view the underside.

2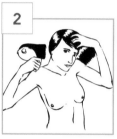
Thoroughly inspect your scalp, using a blow-dryer and mirror to expose each section to view. Get a friend or family member to help, if you can.

6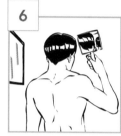
With your back to the full-length mirror, use the hand mirror to inspect the back of your neck, shoulders, upper back, and any part of the back of your upper arms you could not view in step 4.

3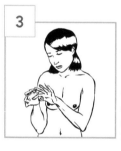
Check your hands carefully: palms and backs, between the fingers, and under the fingernails. Continue up the wrists to examine both front and back of your forearms.

7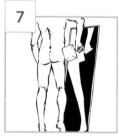
Still using both mirrors, scan your lower back, buttocks, and backs of both legs.

4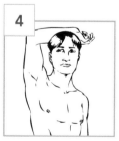
Standing in front of the full-length mirror, begin at the elbows and scan all sides of your upper arms. Don't forget the underarms.

8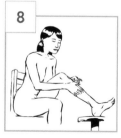
Sit down: prop each leg in turn on the other stool or chair. Use the hand mirror to examine the genitals. Check front and sides of both legs, thigh to shin, ankles, tops of feet, between toes and under toenails. Examine soles of feet and heels.

Understanding Melanoma

3mm

5mm

7mm

9mm

11mm

13mm

15mm

BODY MAP

Mark the position of each mole, freckle, birthmark, bump, or scaly patch you see by making a dot on the body map. (You can draw or photocopy the map if you feel it will be easier to use.)

Draw a line from the dot, and note the date, the size according to the measurement guide at the bottom of the map, and the color.

At each subsequent examination, check each mole for any change in size, color, or shape. Then, add the date and a brief description. Some moles may have appeared since your last examination, and these should be marked on the map and dated.

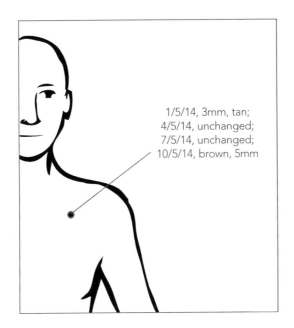

1/5/14, 3mm, tan;
4/5/14, unchanged;
7/5/14, unchanged;
10/5/14, brown, 5mm

DO NOT JUMP TO CONCLUSIONS

If you notice changes in your moles in the course of a self-examination or at any other time, do not immediately assume that you have a melanoma or basal cell or squamous cell carcinoma. Some moles look dangerous, but are benign, while in contrast, some look benign to you, but may be dangerous.

Only a physician can tell one from the other, so if you see a suspicious or unusual mole, make an appointment right away. If the change you observe represents a skin cancer, you can prevent a small problem from developing into a big one.

To be sure not to get off schedule, make up a self-examination calendar, such as this one:

SELF-EXAMINATION SCHEDULE

YEAR 1	YEAR 2	YEAR 3	YEAR 4
Month/Day	Month/Day	Month/Day	Month/Day

See page 36
for instructions.

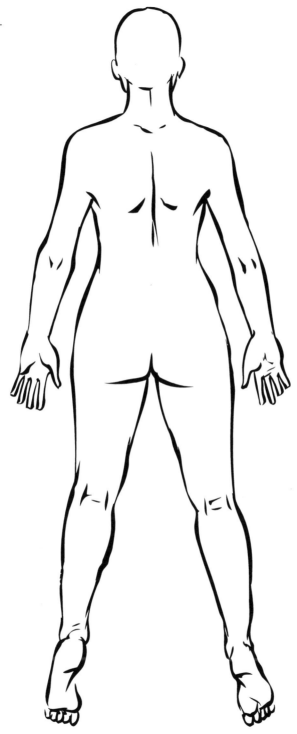

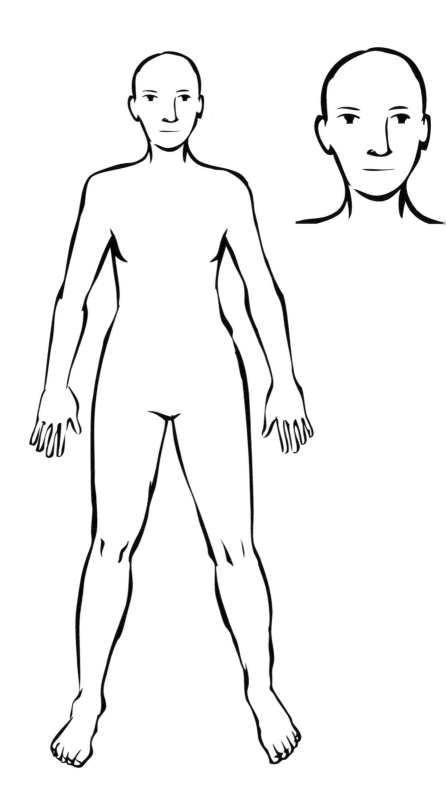

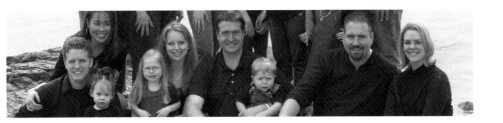

CHAPTER 7

ALL IN THE FAMILY

We are all at risk for melanoma. However, some people are more at risk than others.

Heredity plays a major role. If your mother, father, siblings, or children (first-degree relatives) have had a melanoma, you are part of a melanoma-prone family. Each person with a first-degree relative diagnosed with melanoma has a 50 percent greater chance of developing the disease than members of the general public who do not have a family history of the disease. If the cancer occurred in a grandmother, grandfather, aunt, uncle, niece, or nephew (second-degree relatives), there is still an increase in risk compared to the general population, though it is not as great.

About one of every ten patients diagnosed with the disease has a family member with a history of melanoma.

If melanoma is present in your family, you can protect yourself and your children by being particularly vigilant in watching for the early warning signs and finding the cancer when it is easiest to treat.

Close Relatives Examined

When this skin cancer is diagnosed, it is standard practice for physicians to recommend that close relatives be examined immediately for melanoma and also for the presence of unusual or atypical moles. These moles were formerly called "dysplastic nevi," and many professionals still use the term. People with atypical moles are 7 to 27 times more likely to develop melanoma than the general public, and moles of this type are found in about half of all melanoma patients.

An atypical mole displays some or all of the ABCDEs described in Chapter Five as the warning signals for melanoma. To repeat, these are: Asymmetry—two halves do not match; Border—irregular, poorly-defined; Color—most often multicolored in shades varying from tan to dark brown to black, sometimes with red, white, and blue mixed in; Diameter—usually greater than 1/4 inch; and Evolving or changing.

In addition, these moles tend to be flat or only slightly elevated.

However, under the microscope, atypical moles differ from melanomas in that they do not contain cancerous cells. Instead, microscopically, they look like benign moles, with some unusual physical features.

Atypical Mole Syndrome

The "classic" Atypical Mole Syndrome (AMS) has the following three characteristics:

- 100 or more moles

- One or more moles greater than 8 mm (1/3 inch) in diameter

- One or more moles that look unusual

Research has shown that individuals with atypical mole syndrome have a 10 percent lifetime risk of developing melanoma, a far higher risk than for patients without AMS.

Common Moles

Even common moles increase the likelihood of malignancy, provided they are numerous. The greater the total number of moles on the body, the greater the overall danger of developing melanoma, regardless of whether these moles are atypical or normal-appearing. Recent re-

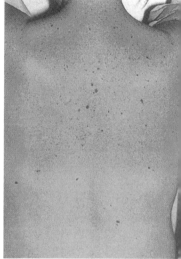

Atypical moles. Upper back was badly sunburned in childhood and has many more moles than lower back.

search shows that having any moles on your body can more than quadruple your risk of developing melanoma. Approximately half of all melanomas develop in preexisting moles. People who have more than 60 moles are 15 times more likely to develop melanoma than are those with no moles, and individuals who have more than 100 moles are at 50 times the risk.

Family Syndrome

When multiple atypical moles (usually 50 or more) are found in an individual belonging to a melanoma family, the condition is known as FAMMM, standing for Familial-Atypical-Multiple-Mole Melanoma Syndrome. People with this form of Atypical Mole Syndrome are at the greatest risk of developing melanoma. In contrast, a research study found that even in melanoma families, individuals who did not have atypical moles were much less likely to develop melanoma.

Genetic Risk Factors

As discussed in chapter 4, about half of all melanoma patients have mutations (alterations) in the BRAF gene, part of the mitogen-activated protein kinase (MAPK) signaling pathway that is involved in both normal physiological and pathological cell proliferation. BRAF is called a "switch" gene, because it turns on to allow cells to grow and divide. When BRAF or other parts of the MAPK pathway such as MEK and NRAS are defective, they can lead to uncontrolled cell growth and promote melanoma. In chapter 4, you can find detailed discussion of the FDA-approved therapies that target the mutant parts of the MAPK pathway to shut down proliferation of melanoma cells.

The mutations most commonly seen in *familial* melanoma occur in another gene, p53, a key regulatory gene . When this gene is in its normal state, its main function is to give damaged cells time to repair themselves and not progress to cancer. However, when the gene is altered, it becomes unable to perform this function, and cancer can result. Complicating matters, new research shows that the same ultraviolet (UV) damage that produces skin damage can damage p53, causing alterations that eliminate its ability to suppress tumors. In contrast, the same research found that skin protected by broad spectrum sunscreen showed no evidence of DNA damage in the keratinocytes, the most common skin cells. These important findings reinforce previous studies demonstrating that sunscreen can help prevent the types of molecular damage induced by sunlight that are known to cause skin cancer.

New research shows that sunscreen can help prevent sunlight-induced molecular damage known to cause skin cancer.

A number of gene mutations in addition to p53 and BRAF have been associated with familial melanoma, notably the CDKN2A (cyclin-dependent kinase inhibitor 2A) gene. In the future, families might be screened to identify those members who are carrying a defective gene. If, as a result, they become particularly vigilant in watching their moles and having regular total-body skin examinations, a melanoma will be detected at its earliest stage when the chances of a cure are excellent. In fact, testing is now commercially available for the presence or absence of the CDKN2A gene, but the consensus of melanoma experts is that genetic testing is not yet warranted for most people and should be done only in the context of clinical trials.

Another "high-risk" melanoma gene, discovered in 2009, is MDM2, which, when mutated and in the presence of estrogen, may increase a woman's propensity for developing melanoma, especially at younger ages. If further research corroborates these findings, it may help explain why younger women have higher melanoma incidence than younger men.

Red-haired variants of the *melanocortin 1 receptor (MC1R)* gene are also associated with an increased risk of melanoma (as well as basal cell carcinoma). MC1R's main function is to determine the type and balance of pigment in the skin, hair, and eyes. While darker-haired, darker-skinned people mainly have a type of melanin called "eumelanin" ("good" melanin) associated with black/brown pigments, redheads predominantly have a type of melanin called "pheomelanin," associated with red/yellow pigments. People who carry the red-hair variants of MC1R have significantly higher risks of melanoma than people who carry the black/brown variants.

Scientists have long known that pheomelanin offers less protection from the sun's ultraviolet rays (UVR) than eumelanin; redheads have no ability to tan and a high susceptibility to rapid sunburn. But new animal research suggests that pheomelanin may not only be less UV-protective, but actually damaging in itself. The researchers compared melanoma incidence in mice with red, albino and dark coat colors, and found that the mice with red coat color had the highest incidence of invasive melanomas, even higher than for the albinos (who have no pigment whatsoever), *even when they had no UV exposure*. The researchers theorized that in the red-haired mice, the intrinsic properties of their pheomelanin were triggering melanomas, like an attack from within. This needs to be confirmed in human studies, but it reinforces the need for redheads to use every means at their disposal to stave off sun damage. Also, since their pigment itself may promote cancer, they need to be acutely aware of any changes in their skin that could herald skin cancer and go in for regular skin exams.

In addition to these mutant genes, certain specific genes involved in the cell cycle may increase melanoma risk when mutated. Each melanoma subtype has its own unique set of mutations. For example, c-Kit and GNAQ mutations are associated with an increased risk of mucosal melanomas and ocular melanomas, respectively. As such genetic variations are discovered, this knowledge will help researchers to design targeted therapies to weaken or nullify the genes' dangerous effects. [See the discussion of targeted therapies in chapter 4.]

Moles in an Active Stage

Moles in people belonging to melanoma-prone families are subject to change at certain times of life. They may grow larger or show alterations in color or elevation, so for those periods, they are described as being active.

While the reasons for these changes are not fully known, there could be a hormonal component: Moles are more active at puberty and during pregnancy. Many — but not all — physicians advise high-risk individuals not to take hormonal medications, such as oral contraceptives or hormone replacement therapy. Therefore, this is a matter to discuss with your doctor.

Examination Scheduling

Individuals with the Atypical Mole Syndrome can improve their chances of early detection by increasing the frequency of skin self-examination and by visiting a physician more often. (Chapter 8 will give you detailed scheduling advice.)

The clinician may take photographs to document whether there are new moles or changes in older ones.

Children: A Special Case

Children in melanoma-prone families need special care, because familial melanoma is likely to make its appearance early in life. Even though these cancers usually do not appear until after adolescence, they may arise in much younger children who have a family history of melanoma. Most physicians, therefore, advise parents to make a point of studying a child's skin frequently from infancy on.

Physician examination should start at the age of ten and continue on a twice-a-year basis thereafter. Particular care should be taken at puberty and during adolescence when hormonal changes activate the moles.

Here is some encouraging news: Because melanoma families are on the lookout for the disease and seek professional consultation early, the survival rate for familial melanoma is even higher than that for nonfamilial melanomas.

CHAPTER 8

GUIDELINES FOR MELANOMA-PRONE FAMILIES

The closer the relationship of the person with melanoma and the greater the number of melanomas in the family, the higher the risk. In addition, many of the relatives who develop melanomas have atypical moles.

As you read in Chapter 7, one of 10 patients diagnosed with melanoma has at least one family member with the disease. Therefore, people belonging to melanoma prone families should protect themselves by observing the following guidelines:

Adults in Families with Atypical Moles and Melanomas

1) Monthly total-body skin self-examination

2) Regularly scheduled total-body skin examination by a physician:

- When moles are stable, they are checked at six-month intervals. A three-month interval is recommended during phases such as puberty, when moles are activated (changing).

- Sometimes pregnant women are evaluated monthly.

3) Minimal sun exposure, particularly when the sun is at its peak from 10 AM to 4 PM

4) Sun-protective clothing:

- Dark-colored or bright-colored, tightly woven fabrics offer the most protection.

- A broad-brimmed hat and sunglasses that block 99 percent or more of ultraviolet rays are essential.

5) Sunscreen:

- Routine use of broad spectrum sunscreens with a Sun Protection Factor (SPF) of 15 or greater for everyday use.

- A broad spectrum water-resistant sunscreen with an SPF of 30 or greater is recommended for extended stays outdoors.

- 1 ounce (2 tablespoons) should be applied to your entire body 30 minutes before going outside so that the sunscreen is fully absorbed by the skin. Reapply every two hours or after swimming or excessive sweating.

6) Avoidance of tanning parlors, sunlamps, sunbeds

7) The potential impact of hormonal medications, such as birth control pills and hormone replacement therapy, should be discussed with the physician.

Children in Families with Atypical Moles and Melanomas

1) Skin examination by parents every two months

2) Physician examination once or twice a year, starting at age ten

3) Sun protection as described for adults

4) Newborns should be kept out of the sun. Sunscreens should be used on babies over the age of six months.

Conclusion: Fewer Melanomas Result

Families that follow these recommendations develop fewer melanomas than those that do not, a National Cancer Institute survey reveals.

What is more, melanomas that do appear are detected more often at the very earliest stage when treatment is easiest and the survival rate is highest.

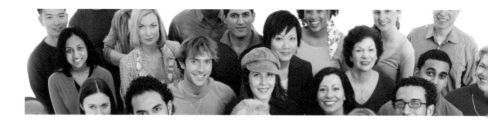

CHAPTER 9

AT RISK FOR MELANOMA

Forewarned is forearmed. Are you at risk for melanoma? If you are and know it you can take steps to reduce that risk.

Some of the major risk factors associated with melanoma are obvious. You have already read about melanoma-prone families and the atypical mole syndrome, but a number of other factors are less well known and may surprise you.

Previous Melanoma

People who have already had a melanoma are five or more times likelier to develop a second than are those who never had one. They are at greatest risk if they also have atypical moles and close relatives with melanoma.

Previous Nonmelanomas

Research also shows that the incidence of melanoma is higher in people with a previous basal cell carcinoma or squamous cell carcinoma (nonmelanomas). The implications are huge, considering that more than 5 million cases of nonmelanoma skin cancer are treated in the US each year.

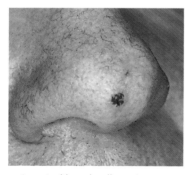

A typical basal cell carcinoma, the most common nonmelanoma skin cancer.

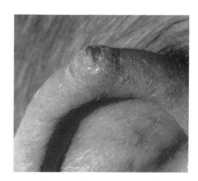

A typical squamous cell carcinoma, also a nonmelanoma skin cancer.

Large Moles in Newborns

Moles that are present at birth or arise shortly thereafter are known as "congenital" moles or "congenital nevi." They are not classified by size at birth, but rather by the size they are expected to be in adulthood:

- small (less than 1.5 cm in diameter),

- medium (1.5-19.9 cm), and

- large (20 cm or larger), sometimes called "giant" nevi.

Any infant with a large congenital mole should be examined by a dermatologist. An estimated 3 to 10 percent of such moles are likely to give rise to melanomas. Fortunately, moles of this type are very rare. When melanomas do occur in these children, approximately 50 percent of them arise during the first three to five years of life.

There is controversy in the medical community about how to treat the congenital moles. Here are the alternatives:

Surgical removal. The entire mole may be excised during the first year of life — at nine to 12 months. However, this requires significant cosmetic repair, and there is no definitive proof that removing a giant congenital mole reduces the overall risk of skin cancer.

Wait-and-see. The physician may instead prefer to watch the mole closely so as to monitor any sudden changes. Surgery is postponed until such changes appear. Some giant moles are simply too large to remove in their entirety.

Small Congenital Moles

If you notice small congenital moles on an infant's body, there is no need to be overly concerned. These do not carry such a high risk of developing into melanoma.

Sun Exposure

The sun's rays are classified according to wavelength, with Ultraviolet B (UVB) being shorter and Ultraviolet A (UVA) longer. Both are dangerous to unprotected skin. UVB produces more intense sunburns, while UVA penetrates the skin to a deeper level, causing premature skin aging (photoaging). Both induce skin cancers, including melanoma. In a landmark 2009 study, scientists at The Wellcome Trust Sanger Institute, in Hinxton, UK, mapped the complete genetic material (the genome) that composed a melanoma taken from a patient with the disease. Using new molecular technology, the researchers identified thousands of mutations, the vast majority of which were caused by UV radiation. Many mutations (changes or errors that occur in genes due to radiation, viruses, and other causes) can ultimately lead to cancer, and this study made perhaps the strongest case ever that some melanomas are indeed caused by exposure to UV radiation.

People who live in locations that have more sunlight — like Florida, Hawaii, and Australia — develop more skin cancers, but some more northern locations with light-skinned populations also have a high number of skin cancers. Avoid using a tanning booth or tanning bed, since it increases your exposure to UV rays, raising your risk of developing melanoma and other skin cancers.

Blistering Sunburns

These are the worst sunburns, indicating excessive sun exposure, and melanomas are found with the greatest frequency in individuals who have experienced them. Severe sunburns do lasting harm to the skin no matter when they occur, but the younger the individual, the greater the risk.

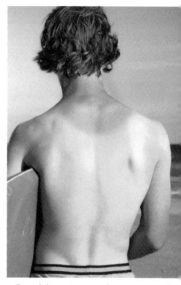

One blistering sunburn in youth more than doubles your lifetime chances of developing melanoma

Childhood

Children should always be protected from the sun, because any sunburn early in life increases the likelihood of melanoma later in life. One blistering sunburn in childhood or adolescence more than doubles a person's chances of developing melanoma later in life.

Until the age of six months, babies should be kept out of direct sunlight altogether their skin may be too sensitive for sunscreen, and contains much less melanin to protect against sun damage. Sunscreen can start being used at six months.

The importance of sun protection cannot be overemphasized, since children spend a substantial amount of time in the sun. Sun safety education should start very early in life.

Equator

In general, people living close to the equator, which has the most intense sun exposure, have the highest incidence of melanoma. This is especially true if the population is light-skinned. Australia is a good example of a sunny, tropical region where most residents are of European descent and have very fair coloring: the number of cases of melanoma there is the highest in the world. One in 25 Australians is likely to develop melanoma over the course of a lifetime, compared to the current US figure of one in 50.

In the US, Hawaii has the greatest incidence of melanoma, even though its population is predominantly dark-skinned. Lentigo maligna, related to chronic sun damage, is the most common form of melanoma seen there.

As discussed, some more northern locations with light-skinned populations also have a high number of skin cancers. One reason may be the tendency to take extended vacations in sunny places, where light skin is extremely vulnerable to sunburn.

Body Sites

Melanomas arise most often in areas frequently exposed to the sun. In Caucasian women, they tend to develop on the legs. When shorter skirts and abbreviated beachwear came into style, the number of melanomas on the legs increased. Caucasian men who remove their shirts for leisure-time activities are most apt to develop these cancers on the back.

However, melanomas also appear often enough on parts of the body normally covered by clothing that total-body skin examination is essential. In general, melanomas on the trunk have been increasing for women as well as men, very possibly due to both outdoor and indoor tanning.

Occasional vs. Continual Sun Exposure

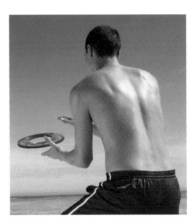

Individuals who are outdoors in intense sunlight only on weekends, vacations, and lunch hours are more prone to melanoma than are those who are continually in the sun. This is especially true when the occasional exposure results in sunburn. Indoor workers, therefore, tend to have melanomas more often than do those whose occupations subject them to the sun's rays throughout the workday. However, everyday outdoor workers have a higher lifetime risk of developing basal and squamous cell carcinoma, the most common nonmelanoma skin cancers.

Artificial Sunlight

Tanning parlors, sunlamps, and sunbeds present an unnecessary and unacceptable risk. They produce ultraviolet radiation that is as or more damaging than natural sunlight; frequent tanners using new high-pressure sunlamps may receive as much as 12 times the annual UVA dose compared to the dose they receive from sun exposure. More than 419,000 cases of skin cancer in the US each year are linked to indoor tanning, including about 245,000 basal cell carcinomas, 168,000 squamous cell carcinomas, and 6,200 melanomas. Recent research has also clearly proven that UV tanning is both physically and psychologically addictive.

In 2009, the International Agency for Research on Cancer, affiliated with the World Health Organization, added UV from indoor tanning to Group One, its list of the most dangerous causes of cancer in humans, alongside other causes such as cigarette smoking, plutonium, and solar UV. In 2014, based on wide-ranging studies detailing the negative health effects of tanning devices, the U.S. Food and Drug Administration reclassified UV tanning lamps from Class I (low to moderate risk) to Class II (moderate to high risk) medical devices. The reclassification enhances FDA regulatory oversight, and requires that a prominent black box warning label be included on every tanning device, including the warning that the device should not be used by persons under age 18.

Eleven states have also forbidden tanning salons to admit patrons under age 18, and many others require parents to give permission for minors to use tanning beds or to accompany them to the tanning salon. There are excellent reasons for keeping young people out of tanning beds, since they are especially vulnerable to lifetime skin damage and increased risk of skin cancer. Of melanoma cases among 18-to 29-year-olds who have tanned indoors, 76 percent are attributable to tanning bed use. People who first use a tanning bed before age 35 increase their lifetime risk for melanoma by 75 percent.

Unfortunately, during the last two decades, the use of tanning parlors has greatly increased, particularly among young women, and women aged 39 and under now have a higher probability of developing melanoma than any other cancer except breast cancer.

Skin Coloring

The fairer the skin, the greater the risk of skin cancer. Melanin, the substance that gives various shades of brown to the skin, also blocks some of the ultraviolet energy from the sun. Nonetheless, this protection is not sufficient, and contrary to what most people believe, dark-skinned peoples do get skin cancer. The numbers, however, are much smaller than for those who are naturally pale. On the other hand, people of color who develop melanoma tend to be diagnosed at a later, more dangerous stage, partly because their cancers can be more aggressive, and partly because their skin is scrutinized for skin cancer less closely.

Classification

Skin is classified according to:

1) the amount of melanin, and

2) the reaction to ultraviolet light exposure.

There are six skin phototypes, going from light to dark. Individuals with skin types I and II are at the highest risk of developing melanomas as well as the other skin cancers, while skin types V and VI face the lowest risk.

To get an idea of the degree of risk you run, rate yourself according to the following classification:

Type I

Very fair, burns easily and severely and does not tan.

Eyes are blue or green and hair is blond.

Type II

Also fair and burns easily, but does develop a minimal tan.

Eyes are blue, hazel, or brown, and hair is blond, red, or brown.

Type III

Somewhat darker and sometimes burns and then tans.

Type IV

Darker still, infrequently burns, and always tans rapidly.

Type V

Brown, tans rapidly and rarely burns.

Type VI

Black, never burns, but is still at risk for skin cancer.

Since anyone — regardless of skin type — can develop melanoma, the need for skin examination and sun protection must never be forgotten.

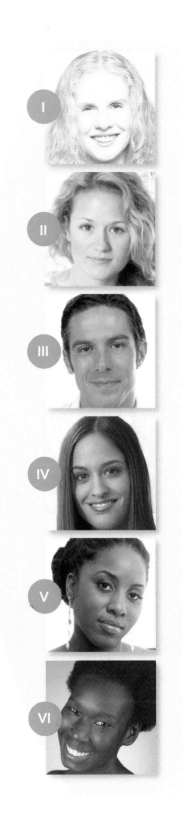

CHAPTER 10

A LOOK AT THE NUMBERS

Melanoma is on the rise and is now the sixth most common cancer in the United States—the *fifth* most common cancer in males. No other cancer is increasing at such a rapid rate; in fact, of the seven most common cancers in the US, melanoma is the only one whose incidence is increasing. In the past 30 years, its incidence has more than tripled.

Lifetime Risk

By 1980, the chance of developing an invasive melanoma over one's lifetime was 1 in 250, quite a change from the 1930s when the risk was 1 in 1,500. It is now 1 in 50. The increase is particularly marked among those under age 40. From 1973 to 2004 in young people age 15 to 39, melanoma incidence increased by 61 percent among males and more than doubled among females. Melanoma is now the most common form of cancer for young adults 25-29 years old and the second most common form of cancer for adolescents and young adults 15-29 years old.

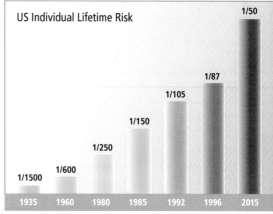

Young women are even more vulnerable than young men; until age 49, they are significantly more likely to develop melanoma than men. Women aged 39 and under now have a higher probability of developing melanoma than any other cancer except breast cancer.

After age 49, men catch up and surpass women. Between ages 60 and 69, nearly twice as many men as women develop this cancer. Overall, it is increasing

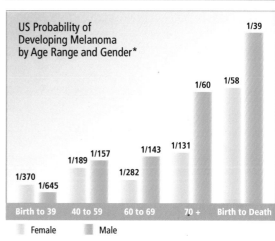

* All sites. Excludes basal and squamous cell skin cancers and *in situ* cancers except urinary/bladder.

Understanding Melanoma

more rapidly than any of the top ten cancers in men. It is also one of only three cancers with an increasing mortality rate for men, along with liver cancer and esophageal cancer.

Incidence and Mortality Statistics

At present, close to 140,000 new cases of melanoma are diagnosed in a year. In 2015, an estimated 73,870 of these will be invasive melanomas, with about 42,670 in males and 31,200 in women. More than 63,000 of the cases will be *in situ* lesions (limited to the top layer of the skin), which are almost always curable if diagnosed early and treated promptly. During the last few years, the incidence of this form of melanoma has increased. In 1999, there were just 23,200 cases, only about 35 percent of today's figure. By the time you read this book, the numbers will probably have climbed even higher.

Although much less common than the nonmelanoma skin cancers (basal cell and squamous cell carcinomas), which strike about 2 million Americans a year, invasive melanoma is far more serious. Melanoma accounts for only about two per-cent of skin cancer cases, but causes the vast majority of skin cancer deaths. An estimated 9,940 melanoma-related deaths—approximately 6,640 men and 3,300 women—will occur in 2015. Almost all will be patients with advanced disease.

Who Gets It

Caucasians

People of all races and skin colors do get cancers, but individuals with fair skin are the most often affected. In fact, according to the most recently available sta-tistics, melanoma rates are more than 25 times higher in Caucasians than in Afri-can-Americans. The incidence of melanomas in Caucasians keeps on rising. From 1973 to 2004 in young Caucasians age 15 to 39, melanoma incidence among males increased by 61 percent and incidence among females more than doubled.

African-Americans

The overall incidence of melanoma has remained steady or decreased among African-Americans. This is attributed to the fact that dark skin contains more of the sun-protective pigment *mela-nin*. However, African-Americans are more likely to be diagnosed at a later stage of the disease than Caucasians, giving them a worse prognosis, partly because their tumors are detected lat-er and partly because they most often develop acral- lentiginous melanoma

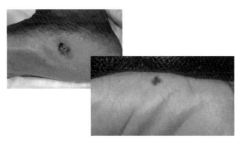

Acral lentiginous melanomas of the feet, legs, and hands are the most common melanomas in African-Americans.

(ALM), a particularly virulent form of melanoma. Their tumors tend to arise in areas not typically exposed to the sun, such as the mucous membranes (mouth, lips, and anogenital areas), palms, soles of the feet, and under the fingernails and toenails. This is also true of Asians, Hawaiians, and Native Americans.

Hispanics

Skin cancer rates among Hispanics are skyrocketing in the US. From 1992 to 2008, their annual melanoma incidence increased by 19 percent. Too little use of sun safety techniques (such as shade, protective clothing, and sunscreen) may have contributed to the rapid rise. In a recent survey, more than 43 percent of Hispanics reported that they never or rarely used sunscreen, only 24 percent said they wear sun-protective clothing, and nearly 40 percent said they sunbathe, with one in three reporting that they sunburned in the past year.

This underuse of sun protection may be partly due to the widespread misconception that people with darker skin are not at risk of skin cancer, to lack of sufficient skin cancer education campaigns targeted to Hispanics, and to the need for physicians to greater emphasize their skin cancer dangers. The truth is, Hispanics vary widely in skin type, from Type 6 (darkest skin) to Type 1 (lightest skin), and while Type 1s are at highest risk of skin cancer, *all* of these are at risk for the disease.

Making matters worse, Hispanics have poorer survival than non-Hispanic patients, often due to later diagnosis. A study in *JAMA Dermatology* found that while 16 percent of initial melanoma diagnoses were late-stage in non-Hispanic white patients, the number jumped to 26 percent for Hispanics. Some of the reasons for later diagnosis are clear: a recent study in North Carolina found that more than three-quarters of Hispanic patients are not performing skin exams and only nine percent receive a regular skin exam from their doctors. For lower income Hispanics, lack of access to medical care contributes to the problem, leaving them with lower skin cancer awareness; this can lead to later diagnosis.

These findings underscore the urgency for year-round sun protection, regular skin self-examination, and annual dermatologist visits for *everyone*, whatever their ethnicity or skin tone.

Hispanics who want to learn more about skin cancer prevention, detection, and treatment can visit The Skin Cancer Foundation's dedicated Spanish language Website, CancerdePiel.org .

Body Sites and Gender

The anatomic site where melanoma tumors are most often located varies according to gender.

Ears. Six times as many men as women develop melanomas on the ears. Their peak age for developing these melanomas is in their eighties.

Legs. Three times as many women as men develop melanomas on the legs. Women in their sixties are at the peak age for tumors at this site. Even so, as men grow older, the number of melanomas on the legs increases.

Face, Scalp, Neck. Twice as many males as females develop melanomas on these sites. Scalp and neck melanomas tend to be especially dangerous; one nationwide study found that people with scalp and neck melanomas die from the disease at nearly twice the rate of people with melanomas elsewhere on the body. Although only six percent of patients have skin lesions on the scalp and neck, they account for 10 percent of all melanoma deaths. One reason for the greater danger of scalp melanomas may be delayed diagnosis due to location, since they are usually hidden by hair and cannot be seen without some effort. The very biology of head and neck melanomas or the environment of the scalp may also play a role. The scalp has numerous blood vessels, and its lymphatic drainage is varied and complex. It may be that melanomas here can more easily spread to the brain, making them more aggressive.

Trunk. While the incidence of melanoma is up at all major body sites, the increase is most marked on the trunk. Here, too, melanomas are found in twice as many men as women. However, more women are developing trunk melanomas than in the past. Also, while men are most likely to be in their sixties when diagnosed, women are more often affected as young as in their thirties.

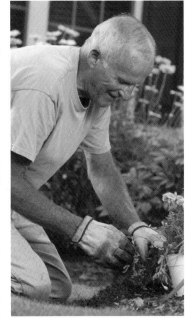

Youth vs. Age

Approximately half of all melanomas occur in individuals younger than 55 years of age, and about 30 percent in those who are younger than 45. However, the largest group of people diagnosed with melanoma are white men over age 50, and between 40 and 50 percent of Americans who live to age 65 will have skin cancer at least once. Caucasian men over age 65 have had a 5.1 percent annual increase in melanoma incidence since 1975, the highest annual increase of any gender or age group.

A key reason for the high skin cancer incidence in people of advanced age is that they are especially vulnerable to the sun's UV rays. This is partly due to all the damage they have already sustained, which keeps adding up over the years; one bad burn in older age may be the straw that broke the camel's back.

Second, senior adults' skin undergoes natural changes that reduce its defenses;

losing fat and water content, it becomes thinner, and is penetrated more deeply by UV than younger skin is.

Third, its ability to repair UV-damaged DNA and correct resulting genetic mutations keeps diminishing. As the mutations increase, so does the risk of skin cancer. Thus, the prevalence of skin disease increases throughout our lives. Most people past 70 have at least one skin problem, and many have three or four. Furthermore, their tumors tend to be larger and more advanced than those in young people, and the outcome of their disease is less often favorable.

Even in older people, though, skin repair processes will more often succeed if an element causing many of the problems is eliminated; namely sun damage. Thus, the older you get, the more essential it is to practice comprehensive sun protection, seeking shade, especially between 10 AM and 4 PM; wearing sun-protective clothing, hats, and UV-blocking sunglasses; and using a sunscreen with an SPF of 30 or higher whenever you're outside. By allowing the skin to rest and recuperate, rather than compounding the damage with further unprotected exposure, older people may avoid many skin cancers.

Melanoma accounts for less than two percent of skin cancer cases, but it causes the vast majority of skin cancer deaths.

It's just as essential for older people to visit a dermatologist regularly. The dermatologist can partially repair some of their lifelong sun damage with lasers and photodynamic therapy, abrasion techniques, and topical medications such as retinoids, not just helping to rejuvenate their skin but also removing some precancerous lesions, thereby reducing their risk of skin cancer. Just as important, the dermatologist can discover cancers at an early stage before they become disfiguring and dangerous.

CHAPTER 11

HOW TO DEVELOP A POSITIVE OUTLOOK

How does someone with melanoma develop a positive, hopeful attitude? It is not easy, but many melanoma patients succeed in doing just that. An optimistic outlook is rewarding both in terms of happiness and in terms of health. People who reject depression and despair have a better chance of being cured.

"I feel very hopeful. I know that I must have a positive attitude and I do have one. I believe that everything I do is the best possible thing. The treatment I'm getting is the best possible treatment for me. I think I made all the right decisions... I'm happy the way things are now."

These words by Richard C. who has endured three recurrences of his disease show how much a positive attitude can mean to a melanoma patient.

TIPS ON COPING SUCCESSFULLY

Here are suggestions on how to live with melanoma. They have worked for many people and may work for you.

- Accept your doubts, fears, and anxiety as normal reactions to cancer. Do not keep these feelings to yourself. Speak first of all to your physician, who is in a position to allay many fears and to put others in perspective. Make a list of the questions you want to ask and bring it to the doctor's office. Check it before leaving so as to be sure that everything troubling you has been discussed.

- Rather than retreating into solitude, reveal your feelings and concerns to family and friends. When appropriate, let them participate in the decisions being made. Welcome their support and interest in you. Marriages and other relationships are frequently strengthened when people face an illness together.

- If, like millions of Americans, you live alone, use the telephone, text messages, email, or social media such as Facebook and Twitter to connect you to family and friends who are far away; consider talking with a colleague, teacher, or religious leader. You can also find Internet groups of other people battling melanoma to share your concerns and learn important new information.

- Relaxation is a tried-and-true method of relieving stress, and everyone can benefit from it. Many tapes, CDs and DVDs that give relaxation techniques are available.

- Devote some time each day to positive imagery—the recollection of a happy experience, the face of someone you love, the beauty of a landscape at sunset or any other thought that gives you pleasure.

- Humor can help create an upbeat feeling. Look for it in books, cartoons, movies, television, and on the Internet.

- Exercise does more than keep you fit: It releases "endorphins." These are brain chemicals that resemble morphine in their ability to lift the mood. Consult your physician about just what kinds of exercise will be good for you.

- Sex can continue to be a part of your life. Do not give up on sexual activity just because of melanoma. Skin cancer is not contagious! Should physical problems arise as a result of the disease or its therapy, discuss them with your physician. Similarly, express feelings of depression, anxiety, or the concern that treatment-induced alterations in appearance will change a partner's attitude. These changes often matter much less to a spouse or friend than the patient thinks they do. You are still the same person; cancer does not alter that.

- Keep up your appearance; it helps to keep up your spirits. Do not stop using cosmetics or shaving; select clothing that is becoming to you. If therapy could cause hair loss, consider obtaining a wig in advance.

- Be good to yourself. Accept the fact that you may tire more rapidly than you did before. If you do not feel your best, do not drive yourself to perform all your former duties. Instead, concentrate on the things you enjoy.

"Get Involved in Living"

"I can extend my life—whether by five years or a day—by getting actively involved in living," says melanoma patient Richard C.

That is the secret to coping with the disease successfully. Rather than looking backwards, look ahead to vacations, career plans, a son's or daughter's graduation from college, or your own.

The Danger of Ignoring Warning Signals

Richard C.'s story begins like those of many melanoma patients with a dark spot that was overlooked, even as it grew larger and darker. Only when it started to bleed did he go to a dermatologist. By then, the melanoma was deeply invasive and extensive surgery was required. A year afterwards came the first recurrence and a second surgery.

The oncologist put Richard C.'s chance of surviving for five years at 20 percent and told him that standard chemotherapy would not help. After discussion with his wife, children, and physician, he decided to enter an immunotherapy program. While he was receiving treatment, he joined the melanoma support group at the medical center. A year later, after yet another recurrence, he found another support group closer to his home.

Support Groups Can Help

Richard C. credits support groups with helping him achieve his positive outlook. He believes that talking to other people with cancer keeps him from feeling alone in the battle against melanoma. "Every time I go to a group meeting, I leave there feeling better," he reports.

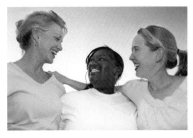

The encouragement you can receive from groups as well as family, friends, and your physician affects the course of the disease favorably. Studies have shown that people with serious illnesses respond better to treatment and live longer when they get emotional support.

If you are being treated at a cancer center, hospital, or medical center, be sure to ask if they have a support group for their patients. Many of them do. In addition, a number of national organizations provide support services. A special list has been compiled for readers of *UNDERSTANDING MELANOMA*, and can be found in Chapter 14.

Do It Yourself

Some melanoma patients have set up support networks themselves. This is the way Sharon P. describes how the newsletter, *The Helping Hand,* was started:

"Six or seven of us sat in the waiting room of the melanoma clinic nervously awaiting our turns for treatment. The silence was unbearable for me, so I started talking about how scared I was. I asked everyone to tell me what they knew about this disease. Instantly the room came alive. All had their own stories, their own fears, and their own dreams of remission and cure."

This small group decided to establish a newsletter and a network to share information and to bring hope and courage to one another. *The Helping Hand* provided facts on treatments, research discoveries, personal experiences, and related reading. "We as a group focused on learning to adapt to a life that included cancer," says

> "Having cancer doesn't change you... unless you let it."

Sharon P. "The knowledge that we were not alone helped us to put fear and uncertainty into perspective."

Sharon P. recalls that the first few months after learning of her cancer were filled with fear, panic, and loneliness. A young woman herself, she felt isolated from others her own age. Then came *The Helping Hand*. "This kind of support is in many ways responsible for my own well-being."

As melanoma survivor Barbara B. sums it up: "Having cancer does not change you . . . unless you let it."

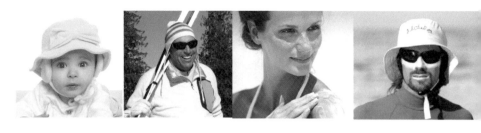

CHAPTER 12

SAFE IN THE SUN

Obviously, it is better to prevent skin cancers than to find and treat them. Yet many of the risk factors for melanoma described in the preceding chapters are beyond your control. You cannot choose the family of your birth, the number of moles you are born with, or your basic skin coloring. But one thing you can change is your exposure to the sun's damaging rays.

SUN PROTECTION TIPS

Follow these sun protection tips whenever you are outdoors:

Clothing

Keep covered. Wear long-sleeved shirts and pants; add a broad-brimmed hat and sunglasses that block 99 percent or more of UVB and UVA. Ideally, your sunglasses should also guard against *High-Energy Visible Light (HEV light)/Blue Light* since HEV light in the violet/blue spectrum is a potential contributor to cataracts and other serious eye maladies.

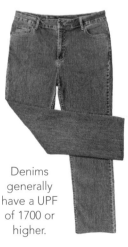

Denims generally have a UPF of 1700 or higher.

Look for tightly woven fabrics. Though most people think white is best, dark and bright colors give better sun protection. So do heavier materials made of fibers such as wool, nylon, silk, polyester, and denim. Today, specially designed clothes with a high *UPF (ultraviolet protection factor)* that can actually wick away sweat and help keep you cool are also available for more measurable protection. UPF indicates how much of the sun's UV radiation is absorbed. A fabric with a UPF rating of 50 will allow only 1/50th of the sun's UV rays to pass through. This means the fabric will reduce your skin's UV radiation exposure significantly, because only 2 percent of UV rays will get through. The Skin Cancer Foundation recommends clothing with a UPF of 30 or higher.

Some clothing, such as white cotton T-shirts, have UPFs as low as 5, and you can suffer a sunburn right through them. So remember to apply sunscreen before getting dressed.

Sunscreen

Apply 1 ounce (2 tablespoons) of sunscreen with a Sun Protection Factor (SPF) of 15 or greater that is "broad spectrum," filtering out both Ultraviolet B (UVB) and Ultraviolet A (UVA). For best results, apply it 30 minutes before going outside so that the skin fully absorbs it, and reapply every two hours or immediately after swimming, bathing, or exercising vigorously. The Skin Cancer Foundation also recommends SPF 30 or higher broad spectrum, water-resistant sunscreens for those with an active outdoor lifestyle or extended stays outdoors.

Two overriding types of sunscreen ingredient exist: chemical sunscreens, which *absorb* the sun's radiation before it can reach the skin, and physical sunscreens such as titanium dioxide and zinc oxide, which literally *deflect* UV rays away from the skin. Since physical sunscreens largely sit atop the skin as a barrier, while chemical sunscreens have to be absorbed into the skin before serving as effective UV absorbers, the physical sunscreens may be safer and less potentially irritating for children and others with sensitive skin.

Shade

Seek the shade, especially during the sun's peak hours of intensity from 10 AM to 4 PM. Take shelter under trees, umbrellas, shade sails, awnings, or gazebos, but remember that not all shade is equally protective. UVB rays can reach the skin indirectly. Indirect or diffuse UV light is radiation that has been scattered by the clouds and other elements in the atmosphere, and/or bounced back from UV-reflective surfaces like dry sand, water, snow, or concrete. A large percentage of the UV light we receive while sitting in the shade is indirect. When you can, seek deep shade, where you cannot see the sky and no UV penetrates.

Sunburn. Do not burn. On average, a person's risk for melanoma doubles if he or she has had more than five lifetime sunburns.

Children

Infants below the age of six months should not be in direct sunlight. Sunscreens are not recommended for their sensitive skin. After the age of six months, sunscreens can be used along with the other sun-protective practices.

Examination. Examine your skin from head to toe once a month, using a full-length mirror and a hand mirror to see the back portions of your body. Use a blow-dryer to help check your scalp.

Tanning. Avoid tanning and never use UV tanning salons. Individuals who have used tanning beds 10 or more times in their lives have a 34 percent increased ris of developing melanoma compared to those who have never used tanning beds.

THE UV INDEX

To help you evaluate the risk on any given day, many television and radio stations newspapers, and the Internet now provide information about the UV (ultraviolet Index. This was developed by the National Oceanic and Atmospheric Administration, the Environmental Protection Agency, and the Centers for Disease Control and Prevention and was actively promoted by public health organizations, including The Skin Cancer Foundation.

The UV Index is an estimate of the peak amount of ultraviolet rays that will reach the earth's surface at "solar noon," the moment of the day with the most intense solar radiation. It is based on day-to-day fluctuations in the stratospheric ozone layer that shields the earth from the sun's rays. The higher the UV Index on a given day, the more intense the sun's UV rays reaching earth are that day.

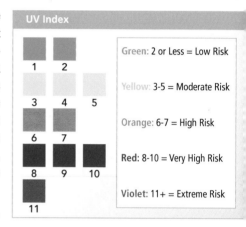

One example of a UV Index chart.

The Skin Cancer Foundation recommends that you always use proper sun protection, regardless of the number on the UV Index.

NO TAN IS SAFE

For most of the 20th century, a tan was considered fashionable, equated with beauty, health, general attractiveness, and affluence. In the 21st century, that view is no longer in style. Today, following the widespread education campaigns carried to the public by The Skin Cancer Foundation and other health organizations, a growing number of Americans know that a tan is the result of DNA damage, and the first step towards skin cancer. It is also a sure cause of wrinkles and other signs of skin aging: More than 90 percent of the visible changes commonly attributed to skin aging are caused by the sun. The Foundation advises everyone to "Go with Your Own Glow"—appreciate and embrace your natural skin color, rather than attempting to darken it by tanning.

**There is no such thing as a safe tan,
so protect yourself from the sun's rays.**

CHAPTER 13

WHAT YOU WANT TO KNOW ABOUT MELANOMA

ANSWERS TO THE 25 QUESTIONS MOST FREQUENTLY ASKED

Q: What is melanoma?

A: Melanoma is a malignant tumor of melanocytes, the pigment-producing cells of the skin. Moles, on the other hand, are benign tumors of melanocytes.

Q. How can it be detected at an early stage?

A: Examine the skin over your entire body so as to spot the first signs of melanoma; if anything looks suspicious, see a physician immediately. Self-examination of the skin should be performed every month and total-body physician skin examination every year.

Anyone who has had a melanoma or possesses another high-risk factor needs to increase the frequency of skin examination. If you fall into this category, ask your physician just how often an exam is advisable.

Q. What are the first warning signs?

A. The five early warning signs of melanoma are known as the ABCDEs: A for Asymmetry—the two sides of the mole do not match; B for Border—the shape is irregular; C for Color—a variety of shades; D for Diameter—usually larger than 6 mm or one-fourth inch; and E for Evolving (changing). Also, watch for danger signals in moles such as increased elevation, scaliness, oozing, itching, or tenderness.

When you observe changes in moles, when new ones appear after the age of 25, or when a mole looks or feels different than all other moles around it (the "ugly duckling" sign), consult a physician right away.

Q. How is a biopsy performed?

A. A biopsy is an important diagnostic test performed when a mole or skin lesion looks suspicious. In this procedure, a piece of tissue is removed surgically and sent to the laboratory, where it is tested for malignancy.

Q. What are the causes?

A. The causes most often cited are heredity (genetic makeup), sun exposure, an indoor tanning. Melanoma is more common in people living in regions that ar comparatively close to the equator: for example, Australia and Hawaii. Some stud ies suggest that risk is increased when a person moves from a northern region t an area that has more intense sun exposure. However, the role of sunlight is no always clear-cut. Inhabitants of areas without much sunshine may develop mela nomas anyway, and sometimes the tumors appear on parts of the body that ar usually covered.

Q. Who is most at risk?

A. Melanoma runs in families, so those whose closest relatives have or have ha melanoma are at higher risk than the general population. Therefore, a total-bod skin examination should be performed by a physician as soon as melanoma i diagnosed in a family member, and should be followed by regular skin self-ex aminations. This is particularly true when many atypical, unusual-looking mole are present, and even people with many *normal* moles are at increased risk. A fai complexion, blue eyes, and blond hair add to the susceptibility, as does a histor of sunburns.

Q. Is melanoma contagious?

A. No. Melanoma cannot be transmitted by contact. This means that you canno "catch" melanoma from a family member or friend. The prevalence of this cance in families is due to an inherited gene, not contagion.

Q. When is a melanoma "advanced?"

A. Early-stage melanomas either have not penetrated the skin (*in situ*, stage 0) o remain small, nonulcerated, and confined to the primary tumor in the top layers o the skin (stage 1). Melanoma is considered advanced when it spreads, or metasta sizes, beyond the primary tumor to other sites. The cancerous cells may enter th lymph nodes close to the original tumor and/or may be passed through the lymp fluid or bloodstream to more distant nodes.

At its most advanced stage, the melanoma has traveled via the bloodstream to in vade internal organs, such as the lung, liver, brain, or bone.

Q. How are metastases recognized?

A. First, it is known that a melanoma is more likely to spread if it is thick and ha penetrated deeply into the skin; if it is ulcerated (open and bleeding) or has a high mitotic rate (rapid growth rate), it is even more likely to metastasize. In each o these cases, the physician will feel the lymph nodes near the tumor for lumps o swellings, and will also most likely do a sentinel node biopsy to see if the tumo has spread to the local lymph nodes. The liver and spleen will also be checked.

A number of diagnostic tests can be done when distant metastasis—disease spread beyond the local lymph nodes—is suspected. These include blood tests, chest x-ray, CT (computed tomography) imaging scans, MRI (magnetic resonance imaging) scans, PET (positron emission tomography) scans, or other studies.

Q. What are the main treatments in use today?

A. In the early stages, the treatment for melanoma is surgical removal alone, and the results are almost always excellent; average 5-year survival is 98 percent. If the tumor is larger or has other high-risk factors for metastasis, the nearby lymph nodes may also be examined; generally a sentinel node biopsy will first be done to see if the cancer has reached the lymph nodes. If the sentinel nodes (the first nodes into which the tumor drains) prove negative for cancer, the surgery ends. If the cancer has reached the sentinel nodes, the rest of the nodes in that local nodal basin will all be removed. If the tumor has spread, immunotherapy and/or targeted therapy and chemotherapy might be added, generally taken orally or injected intravenously.

Q. What is immunotherapy?

A. This is a form of treatment aimed at strengthening the patient's immune system so that it is better able to fight off the tumor when a patient has reached Stage II or higher. Immunotherapy may be combined with other treatments, including standard surgery and/or chemotherapy or targeted therapy.

There are several types of immunotherapies utilizing mass-produced versions of chemicals that occur naturally in the body. For Stage II and III patients, high-dose interferon alfa-2b (IFN-alfa-2b) has been the most widely used FDA-approved treatment, while high-dose interleukin-2 (IL-2) is the longest-used FDA-approved treatment for Stage IV patients. These drugs have slowed the disease down and delayed recurrence, but have had limited results in extending long-term survival for most patients.

In 2011, the FDA approved peginterferon alfa-2b (also known as Sylatron™), a modified version of high-dose IFN-alpha-2b, to treat Stage III patients. Injected subcutaneously, it is the first adjuvant, or additional, therapy for Stage III patients approved since high-dose IFN alfa-2b in 1995, but while it may delay recurrence, it has not been found to increase overall survival.

In the past few years, however, a major revolution has occurred in immunotherapy for advanced melanoma patients. Today, the most exciting new immunotherapies are the "checkpoint blockade" therapies. The first successful checkpoint blockade therapy was ipilimumab (Yervoy™), approved by the FDA in 2011 for patients with advanced melanoma. A monoclonal antibody (a purified class of antibodies cloned and mass-produced in the lab from one specific type of cell or cell line), it blocks CTLA-4, which is a kind of natural "brake" in the immune system that can inhibit activation of healing T-cells. Ipilimumab binds to CTLA-4 so that the T-cells can once again be released to naturally treat the melanoma. It has yielded dramatic, sustained responses akin to "cures" in certain patients, with some surviving more than 5 or even 10 years.

In 2014, two drugs in a new class of checkpoint blockers were FDA-approved for metastatic melanoma patients: pembrolizumab (Keytruda®) and nivolumab (Opdivo®). Both inhibit another molecule called programmed death-1, or PD-1, which like CTLA-4 suppresses T-cells. Both drugs bind up PD-1 so that it can no longer keep the T-cells from fighting the melanoma. These drugs are used when ipilimumab treatment has failed, and to date they appear to be even more effective than ipilimumab. They could in the near future become front-line therapies.

Q. What is the status of vaccines?

A. Immunotherapy also includes the use of vaccines made with melanoma cells taken from the person being treated or from other melanoma patients. Quite a number of different vaccines have been developed and have undergone or are undergoing clinical testing at many major medical centers.

There is some evidence that vaccines slow the progression of melanoma in certain patients, but these treatments are still experimental, and to date they have shown no survival advantage.

Q. How is gene therapy used?

A. The goal is to alter selected genes to correct genetic defects or enhance the cancer-fighting potential of cells. In one form of gene therapy, the patient's own immune cells from the blood (e.g., lymphocyte-activated killer cells) or from the tumor (tumor-infiltrating lymphocytes) are removed, grown, and expanded in number outside the body. Then genetic material is added to produce growth factors that make the lymphocytes or killer cells more aggressive. These more aggressive lymphocytes are returned to the patient's body in an effort to stimulate the immune system to attack the melanoma and its metastases. This therapy is still experimental, but studies to date have had promising results.

Another type of gene therapy targets genes like BRAF and MEK, which when defective turn into cancer-producing genes. Their defective proteins get stuck in the "on" position, allowing uncontrolled cell growth, and treatments like vemurafenib dabrafenib, and trametinib bind up or block those proteins, turning off the uncontrolled growth and thus correcting the defective gene for a certain period of time.

In the future, scientists hope also to alter inherited mutant versions of genes such as CDKN2A (p16) and the so-called "redhaired" variants of the melanocortin 1 receptor gene (MC1R), which are passed from generation to generation in certain families or ethnic groups, leaving family members at high risk of developing melanoma. Yet another focus of research is identifying genes for specific melanoma antigens that stimulate production of antibodies. By injecting the genes for these melanoma antigens, the hope is to increase their number and produce a broad attack by the patient's immune system. But all of these treatments are in very early stages of research.

Q. Should a cancer specialist be consulted?

A. Your regular physician or dermatologist will make a recommendation as to whether an oncologist should be consulted. Usually, the decision on how to proceed depends on the likelihood of spread.

Q. What are the chances of having another melanoma?

A. People who have had one melanoma are at higher risk of developing a second. Therefore, they are usually advised to have regular check-ups by a physician every three months for two years, every six months for three more years, and then yearly for life. The doctor will watch for signs of recurrence at the site of the original tumor, check for the presence of unusual moles, evaluate the lymph nodes, investigate the subcutaneous tissue, and look for distant organ involvement.

Q. Are subsequent melanomas treated differently from the first?

A. That depends on whether they are different. In all cases, treatment is based on the thickness and depth of invasion of the tumor and whether it has spread. As patients who have had one melanoma are given frequent check-ups, second primary (new, localized) melanomas can be caught at an early stage and treated by surgical excision. However, melanoma *recurrences* are often discovered at an advanced stage and can be extremely dangerous.

Q. Should hormones be avoided?

A. The advisability of taking hormones, such as optional oral contraceptives or hormone replacement therapy, is controversial. Some doctors believe that in patients with a history of melanoma, hormones can stimulate new melanoma development, while others feel there is no effect.

The risks shown by recent studies to be associated with hormone replacement therapy also have to be weighed against the potential benefit for those at high risk of osteoporosis.

Q. Is pregnancy a problem?

A. The influence of pregnancy on the course of melanoma is debatable. A number of studies show that pregnancy does not affect localized State I or II melanomas, the kind found in most women. But more uncertainty comes with advanced melanomas.

Q. Does pregnancy change the course of advanced disease?

A. Controversy exists about the effect of pregnancy on more advanced disease with some evidence indicating that metastatic melanoma during pregnancy can be particularly aggressive. However, though moles commonly become larger and darker during pregnancy due to increased levels of estrogen and melanocyte-stimulating hormone, no conclusive evidence exists that pregnancy significantly increases the incidence of metastasis or lowers overall survival. Thus, terminating the pregnancy of a newly diagnosed melanoma patient as a therapeutic measure cannot currently be recommended.

On the other hand, melanoma is one of the most common tumors known to metastasize to the placenta and fetus, so the child will have to be monitored carefully for melanoma after birth. Furthermore, if the disease is diagnosed during pregnancy it must be treated, and unfortunately, both diagnosis and treatment of melanoma from Stage II on may be problematic for the fetus. The radioactive tracers used in sentinel node biopsy mapping and imaging techniques such as PET-scans and CT scans which employ radiation may be harmful to the fetus, as are treatments for advanced disease such as vemurafenib.

Q. What advice is given to patients who want to become pregnant?

Since the vast majority of recurrences occur within 2-3 years after treatment of the primary lesion, many women are advised to postpone pregnancy for a minimum of two years after the initial diagnosis of an early melanoma. This is a precaution based on the uncertainty about the effect of pregnancy on melanoma.

If the malignancy has spread to the lymph nodes or distant organs, most physicians will advise against becoming pregnant altogether.

Q. Is there a special melanoma diet?

A. No, but patients who are in good health, aside from the cancer, are always likely to have a better response to treatment if they follow sound nutritional practices. They should make a point of consuming a balanced diet that provides sufficient calories, protein, and nutrients to maintain body weight. Vitamins and minerals are important, especially folic acid; vitamins B-6, B-12, C, and A; iron, and zinc.

Q. Should patients avoid the sun?

A. The Skin Cancer Foundation recommends that all people, including melanoma patients, protect themselves from the sun whenever they are outdoors. While there is no evidence that sun exposure will change the course of an existing melanoma, it may increase the risk of developing another. It can also cause nonmelanoma skin cancers, primarily basal cell carcinomas (BCCs), and squamous cell carcinomas (SCCs).

Therefore, it is important to minimize exposure from 10 AM to 4 PM when the sun is at its peak; wear protective clothing, including a broad-brimmed hat and sunglasses that block 99 percent or more of UV rays; and use a sunscreen with an SPF of 15 or greater [SPF 30 or higher for extended stays outdoors].

Q. Is it safe to donate blood?

A. Most blood centers do not accept blood from anyone who has had cancer.

Q. Where can I get more information?

A. You can obtain brochures on melanoma, other skin cancers, and sun protection tips by visiting The Skin Cancer Foundation's Website at SkinCancer.org. See Appendix B in this book for a list of available materials.

Q. How can I join The Skin Cancer Foundation?

A. For membership information, contact The Skin Cancer Foundation: E-mail: development@skincancer.org, or visit our Website at SkinCancer.org.

CHAPTER 14

GUIDE TO INFORMATION SOURCES and SUPPORT GROUPS

Support services give not only information, but also encouragement and hope. There are many more than can possibly be listed here. The support groups and sources presented in this chapter have been specially selected for *UNDERSTANDING MELANOMA*.

In addition, many cancer centers, hospitals, and medical centers maintain support groups for their patients and family members, or suggest places to go. Ask your doctor or local hospital whether such a group is available near you.

The Skin Cancer Foundation

The only international organization devoted exclusively to educating the public and medical professionals about skin cancer prevention, detection and treatment. Our website, SkinCancer.org, along with its Spanish-language version, Cancerde Piel.org, is the world's leading online source for skin cancer information. In addition, we publish brochures, newsletters, an annual journal, posters, books, and classroom curriculums, with publications available in seven different languages. A "Physician Finder" listing is offered on the website. Public and professional education campaigns are conducted in the US and abroad, and the Road to Healthy Skin tour provides free skin cancer screenings across the country. The Foundation also offers certain grants to researchers working on treatments for melanoma.

149 Madison Avenue, Suite 901• New York, NY 10016 • info@skincancer.org • SkinCancer.org

American Academy of Dermatology (AAD)

With a membership of more than 17,000 physicians worldwide, the AAD is committed to raising awareness of all skin, hair and nail conditions, including melanoma. Their SPOT Skin Cancer program uses public awareness, community outreach, free public skin cancer screenings and other services to promote the prevention, detection and care of skin cancer. To find a dermatologist and to access information and resources on skin cancer prevention and detection, visit SpotSkinCancer.org.

P.O. Box 4014 • Schaumburg, IL 60618-4014
1-866-503-SKIN • T: 1-847-240-1280 • mrc@aad.org • aad.org

American Cancer Society

A major source for information on cancer treatment, medicine, pain control, clinical trials, and referrals for emotional and financial support. Trained cancer treatment specialists are available 24 hours a day on a free hotline. Gives support to patients, survivors and caregivers.

250 Williams Street NW • Atlanta, GA 30303
1-800-227-2345 • cancer.org

American Childhood Cancer Organization

A nationwide organization that offers support and advocacy for families of children with cancer, survivors of childhood cancer, and the professionals who care for them. Informative books for adults and children are provided free of charge to those with financial constraints.

P.O. Box 498 • Kensington, MD 20895-0498
855-858-2226 • T: 301-962-3520 • Staff@acco.org • acco.org

American Melanoma Foundation

Maintains an online listing of support groups and advises anyone wanting to start one. Gives information about melanoma from screening to staging, including clinical trials that patients may wish to join.

4150 Regents Park Row, Suite 300 • El Cajon, CA 92020

T: 619-448-0991 • melanomafoundation.org

Angel Flight America

Patients needing medical care at distant locations receive free flights from these volunteer pilots. Primarily serves the heartland region.

Tulsa, OK 74128

T: 918-749-8992• F: 918-745-0879

angel@angelflight.com • angelflight.com

Association of Cancer Online Resources (ACOR)

A collection of 142 cancer-related email lists providing information and support for patients, caregivers and friends, including an online community for melanoma patients and survivors.

173 Duane Street, Suite 3A • New York, NY 10013

T: 1-212-226-5525 • acor.org

Cancer Care Inc.

Offers free, professional support services for cancer patients and families, by phone, online and in person through support groups. Call their toll-free "Cancer Care Counseling Line" to be connected with resources.

275 7th Avenue, 22nd Floor. • New York, NY 10001

1-800-813-HOPE • T: 212-712-8400 • info@cancercare.org • cancercare.org

Cancer Hope Network

Patients and family members are matched with cancer survivors who serve as mentors, supporting them through the treatment process.

2 North Road, Suite A • Chester, NJ 07930

1-800-552-4366 • T: 908-879-4039

info@cancerhopenetwork.org • cancerhopenetwork.org

Cancer Support Community

In 2009, the Wellness Community and Gilda's Club Worldwide merged to form the Cancer Support Community, an international non-profit devoted to helping cancer patients through counseling, support groups, and healthy lifestyle programs. Check online for local affiliate groups.

1050 17th Street, NW Suite 500 • Washington, DC, 20036

1-888-793-9355 • T: 202-659-9709 •

help@cancersupportcommunity.org • cancersupportcommunity.org

The Candlelighters® Childhood Cancer Family Alliance

A nationwide organization offering support and advocacy to families of children with cancer, survivors of childhood cancer, and the professionals who care for them. Informative books are provided free of charge to those with financial constraints.

8323 Southwest Freeway, Suite 435 • Houston, Texas 77074

T: 713-270-4700 • gfoust@candle.org • Candle.org

Caregivers Action Network (CAN)

Formerly the National Family Caregivers Association, CAN provides education peer support and resources to family caregivers across the country.

1130 Connecticut Avenue NW, Suite 300• Washington, DC 20036

202-454- 3970 • info@caregiveraction.org • caregiveraction.org

Corporate Angel Network

Cancer patients traveling long distances for treatments can fly for free on vacant seats on corporate jets.

Westchester County Airport • 1 Loop Road• White Plains, NY 10604

T: 914-328-1313 • info@corpangelnetwork.org • corpangelnetwork.org

Hill-Burton Free Hospital Care

A federal law mandating certain hospitals to provide free or reduced-cost health care to those who can't afford to pay. Check online or call their hotline for a list of Hill-Burton obligated facilities.

1-800-638-0742 • 1-800-492-0359 (for Maryland residents) • hrsa.gov

Look Good...Feel Better

Provides makeovers and beauty consultations for people undergoing cancer treatments. Founded by the Personal Care Products Council Foundation, the American Cancer Society, and the Professional Beauty Association.

1-800-395-LOOK • lookgoodfeelbetter.org

Make-A-Wish Foundation® of America

An organization that grants wishes for children battling life-threatening illnesses. Local chapters can be found throughout the US and internationally.

4742 N. 24th St., Suite 400 • Phoenix, AZ 85016

1-800-722-WISH • T: 602-279-WISH • mawfa@wish.org • wish.org

Melanoma International Foundation

An organization devoted to supporting melanoma patients as they navigate the treatment process. Their website includes information on understanding pathology reports, prognosis, therapy options and the latest in clinical trials.

250 Mapleflower Road • Glenmoore, PA 19343

T: 866-463-6663 • contact@melanomainternational.org• melanomaintl.org

Melanoma Research Foundation (MRF)

Supports research for effective treatments and eventually a cure for melanoma, through grant funding to established investigators, research teams, and junior investigators. Educates patients, families, caregivers and the medical profession about the prevention, diagnosis, and treatment of melanoma. Acts as an **advocate** for the melanoma community to raise awareness of this disease and the need for a cure. Its online forum, the Melanoma Patients Information Page (MPIP), provides patients, caregivers, family and friends with a space to share information and support one another. Its Cure OM Forum is a space for patients and caregivers affected by ocular melanoma, and its Chat Room is a peer-connection space for patients and caregivers affected by melanoma.

1411 K Street, NW Suite 800• Washington, DC 20005

800-673-1290 • Helpline 877-673-6460 • Melanoma.org

National Cancer Institute (NCI)

A division of the National Institutes of Health, this federal agency coordinates all cancer-related activities. Its website is a good information source on cancer treatments, clinical trials, and cancer centers. The agency has a toll-free information line and live help online.

BG 9609 MSC 9760• 9609 Medical Center Drive • Bethesda, MD 20892

1-800-4-CANCER • cancer.gov

National Coalition for Cancer Survivorship

An advocacy organization for cancer patients and survivors working to improve the quality of life and care for the millions affected by the disease. The Coalition offers Cancer Tool Box, a free audio program encouraging cancer patients to take a more active role in their care.

1010 Wayne Avenue, Suite 315• Silver Spring, MD 20910

1-877-NCCS-YES (622-7937) • T: 301-650-9127 •

info@canceradvocacy.org • www.canceradvocacy.org

Oncolink

An online information resource for both patients and health professionals on available cancer treatments, the latest research, and how to find support. Founded by UPENN Medicine. Oncolink.org

Partnership for Prescription Assistance

A program funded by pharmaceutical companies, it helps qualifying patients get free or low-cost drug prescriptions. pparx.org

Patient Access Network (PAN) Foundation

Helps the underinsured with chronic or life-threatening conditions to pay for treatment and prescription drugs. Has funds set aside specifically for melanoma patients.

PO Box 221858 • Charlotte, NC 28222

866-316-PANF (7263) • contact@panfoundation.org • panfoundation.org

Patient Advocate Foundation

Provides free case managers to serve as a liaison between patients and insurers, employers and creditors. Advocates on behalf of patients so that they can obtain access to care, keep their jobs and be financially stable.

421 Butler Farm Rd. • Hampton, VA 23666

1-800-532-5274 • help@patientadvocate.org • patientadvocate.org

Vital Options®

A cancer support organization and founder of The Group Room®, formerly a nationally syndicated cancer radio talk show that has now fully transitioned to a video website, facilitating a global cancer dialogue.

• T: 818-508-5657 • info@vitaloptions.org • www.vitaloptions.org

GLOSSARY

ABCDEs of melanoma – An acronym for the five most basic warning signs that a mole may be a melanoma: **A**symmetry; **B**order irregularity; **C**olor variability **D**iameter over six millimeters (1/4 inch), and **E**volving or changing.

Acral lentiginous melanoma – An often virulent form of melanoma that arises on the palms, soles, under the nails, or on the mucous membranes. The most common type of melanoma in African-Americans and Asians.

Actinic keratosis – The most common potentially precancerous skin lesion, it appears as a scaly, crusty bump on the skin surface. Also known as "solar keratosis." The plural is "keratoses."

Adoptive cell transfer (ACT) – A treatment technique that involves harvesting tumor-infiltrating lymphocytes (TILs) from a melanoma patient's blood, then isolating from them the cells expressing T cell receptors that can recognize melanoma-specific antigens. These aggressive melanoma-killing cells are then grown in large numbers in the lab and reinjected into the patient with the aim of powerfully attacking the patient's melanoma cells.

Adjuvant therapy – Additional therapy that follows surgery for cancers that have advanced beyond stage I, usually involving chemotherapy, radiation, and/or immunotherapy.

Advanced melanomas – Melanomas that have reached stages III or IV, usually metastasizing to the regional lymph nodes (Stage III) or to distant parts of the body (Stage IV), potentially including vital organs.

Amelanotic melanoma – A type of melanoma that is unpigmented.

Anatomical region or site – A portion or section of the body: for example, the legs arms, or trunk.

Anti-angiogenic therapy – A type of chemotherapy that attempts to kill tumors by preventing new blood vessels from forming, thereby cutting off the blood supply that otherwise nourishes the cancer cells and enables them to grow.

Antibody – A part of the body's defense mechanism formed in response to a foreign antigen. Antibodies attack infectious agents and toxic substances.

Anti-CTLA-4 therapy (also called "checkpoint blockade" therapy) – An important new direction for melanoma immunotherapy. CTLA-4 is a natural "brake" in the immune system that inhibits overactivation of healing T-cells. Anti-CTLA-4 therapies block CTLA-4 so that more T cells can be produced to fight a cancer. The first and best-established of these therapies is ipilimumab (Yervoy®), a monoclonal antibody FDA-approved in 2011 that has had tremendous success with Stage IV melanoma, extending up to 20 percent of patients' lives by 5-10 years or more.

Anti-PD-1 therapy – the newest type of "checkpoint blockade" immunotherapy. PD-1, or programmed cell death-1, is a protein receptor that plays an important role in downregulating the immune system by inhibiting activation of T cells, thereby preventing dangerous autoimmune reactions. Cancers such as melanoma, however, can trick PD-1 and its ligand PD-L1 into inhibiting the T cells, keeping them from attacking the cancer. The new anti-PD-1 therapies inhibit PD-1, thereby reactivating the T cells to fight the cancer. In 2015, the FDA approved two such drugs, pembrolizumab (Keytruda®) and nivolumab (Opdivo®), for Stage IV melanoma patients who have failed treatment with ipilimumab and/or targeted anti-BRAF therapies. These drugs are having even more impressive results than ipilimumab.

Antigen – A molecule found on the cell wall of bacteria, viruses, or tumor cells, it stimulates the body to produce a specific antibody to fight the foreign invader.

Atypical mole – A mole that is unusual in shape, color, and size, often resembling a melanoma, which may indicate that an individual is at increased risk for melanoma. Also known as "dysplastic nevus."

Atypical mole syndrome – A specific condition associated with a highly increased risk of melanoma; the patient has 100 or more atypical moles, one or more moles greater than 8 mm in diameter, and one or more moles that look unusual.

Basal cell carcinoma – The most common form of skin cancer. Made up of cells resembling the basal cells found in the lowest level of the epidermis.

Beauty and the Beast – one of the newer techniques used in dermoscopic analysis of pigmented lesions to help determine if a lesion is melanoma, another malignancy, or a benign growth. In the Beauty and the Beast algorithm, the dermoscopic pattern of the lesion is compared against nine established, typical benign patterns, and if it strays from any of these patterns, a biopsy should be considered.

Benign – Not cancerous; not dangerous to health.

Biopsy – A sample of tissue removed from a mole or skin lesion suspected of being abnormal or cancerous. It is sent to the laboratory for microscopic examination and diagnosis.

Blue-Black Rule – a technique for early recognition that is more sensitive for nodular melanoma than the ABCDEs. It calls attention to any lesion containing some dark blue and black color that doesn't resemble other surrounding lesions.

BRAF – A gene that when mutated can lead to uncontrolled cell growth and cancer, and can play a part in causing melanoma. It is mutated in about half of all melanoma patients. Several FDA-approved drug therapies and combination drug therapies can at least temporarily reverse mutant BRAF's effects and stop uncontrolled melanoma growth for months or years.

Breslow's thickness (also called Breslow's depth) – The measurement in millimeters of the distance between the top layer of the skin and the deepest penetration reached by the melanoma — a key factor in staging early melanomas.

Carcinogen – A chemical or other irritant believed to cause cancer. Examples are soot, charcoal, cigarette smoke, asbestos, and arsenic, as well as exposure to ultraviolet light from sunlight or tanning beds.

Carcinoma – A group of malignant cells that escape normal regulatory systems. These cells may spread from the original site to other parts of the body.

CDKN2A (cyclin-dependent kinase inhibitor 2A) – A key gene associated with familial melanoma.

Checkpoint Blockade Therapy – a type of immunotherapy that inhibits molecules such as CTLA-4 and PD-1, which prevent T cells from attacking melanoma and other cancers. See anti-CTLA-4 therapy and anti-PD-1 therapy.

Chemotherapy – The use of certain drugs, many of them experimental, as additional ("adjuvant") treatments along with surgery to treat advanced cancers and other conditions.

Clark's level – The depth of melanoma penetration, from epidermis in level I to subcutaneous fat in level V. In the newest melanoma staging system, its importance is diminished.

Cobimetinib – an experimental MEK inhibitor that has been tested on BRAF positive advanced melanoma patients, in combination with the BRAF inhibitor vemurafenib. Patients on the combination therapy have lived on average four months longer than on vemurafenib alone. The drug has been submitted to the FDA and could be approved in 2015.

Congenital nevi – Moles that are present at birth or arise shortly after birth. Large congenital nevi (also called giant nevi) often indicate an increased risk of melanoma.

Confocal scanning laser microscopy – This imaging technique makes use of a low-power visible or near-infrared laser, a scanning microscope, and a computer with software to enhance digitized pictures. It allows real-time (in vivo), high-resolution examination of the cellular and sometimes subcellular structures in the epidermis and papillary dermis, before a biopsy is performed. Multiple CSLM units are now available and FDA-approved, including new versions with miniaturized, more user-friendly handheld confocal scanners.

Cryosurgery – A method of treating benign or malignant skin lesions by freezing usually with liquid nitrogen.

CT (computerized tomography) scan (also called computed axial tomography, or CAT, scan) – A high definition type of X ray that examines serial horizontal sections of the body, often the brain, lungs, abdomen, or pelvic cavities.

CUBED Guide for Nail Melanomas – a recently devised guide to early warning signs of nail melanomas, since they differ from the classic ABCDE warning signs. CUBED is an acronym for C=Colored lesions, U=Uncertain diagnosis, B=Bleeding under the nail and the appearance of beefy red tissue, E=Enlargement or deterioration of the lesion or the wound area despite treatment, and D=Delay in healing beyond two months.

Curettage – A method of removing a lesion by scraping it with a special instrument that has a small sharp ring at one end.

Cutaneous – Of or pertaining to the skin.

Dabrafenib (Taflinar®) – an FDA-approved drug that targets and at least temporarily inhibits the mutated BRAF gene in advanced melanoma patients, often stopping uncontrolled melanoma growth for months or sometimes years. In 2014, the FDA also approved its use in combination with a related drug, the MEK inhibitor trametinib (Mekinist™), for patients with inoperable or metastatic melanoma with a BRAF V600E or V600K mutation. Patients on combined dabrafenib and trametinib have been found to have significantly prolonged progression-free survival compared to those on dabrafenib alone.

Dermatologist – A physician who has special training in the diagnosis and treatment of skin conditions and diseases.

Dermatopathologist – A physician who specializes in and has had special training in studying and diagnosing cutaneous diseases at a microscopic and molecular level.

Dermis – The layer of the skin directly below the surface layer (epidermis).

Dermoscope or Dermatoscope – A diagnostic instrument that magnifies the internal structures of a pigmented lesion, helping to distinguish melanomas from other lesions. Formerly, non-polarized dermoscopy (NPD) used non-polarized light that required direct contact with a liquid or gel between the dermoscope and the skin. Today, polarized contact dermoscopy (PCD) and polarized non-contact dermoscopy (PNCD) use cross-polarized light, which does not require the liquid or gel contact. All three techniques can be used as complements to one another to gain extra information.

Desmoplastic melanoma – a variant of melanoma most often associated with lentigo maligna melanoma and the invasive vertical growth phase of a lesion. These unusually fibrous, often nonpigmented tumors may initially appear to be something other than melanoma.

DTIC (dacarbazine) – Given by injection, the only chemotherapy approved by the Food and Drug Administration for Stage IV melanoma.

Dysplastic nevi – Another term for atypical moles.

EFG Rule for Nodular Melanomas – an alternative acronym to the ABCDE rule since nodular melanomas may not be recognizable using the ABCDEs. The EFG acronym stands for **E**levated, **F**irm on palpation, and **G**rowing progressively for over a month.

Electrodesiccation – A treatment for basal and squamous cell carcinoma. Following curettage, an electrically heated needle is used to destroy residual cancer cells and control bleeding.

Epidemiology – The study of the types of diseases, their incidence, distribution and characteristics in a given population.

Epidermis – The top layer of the skin.

Erythema – Redness on the skin, usually produced by blood cells concentrating in an area that is inflamed, infected, or damaged. Sunburn is an example of erythema.

Etiology – The cause or causes of a disease.

Excision – Complete surgical removal of a lesion by cutting it out with a scalpel.

FAMMM (Familial-Atypical-Multiple-Mole Melanoma Syndrome) – The hereditary condition that exists when multiple atypical moles (usually 50 or more) are found in an individual belonging to a melanoma family. It indicates a highly increased risk of melanoma.

Fascia – Thick fibrous tissue that lies beneath the fat and surrounds the muscles.

Gene – The basic hereditary unit that codes the development of the proteins that form the individual and the species.

Gene therapy – A type of therapy that involves altering selected genes to correct genetic defects or enhance the disease-fighting potential of cells.

Guided fine-needle aspiration cytology – a form of ultrasound used before sentinel node biopsy and during follow-up for detection of lymph node metastases. This minimally invasive technique may decrease the need for some SLNBs; patients whose sentinel nodes test positive in ultrasound can proceed straight to radical dissection.

Histology or Histological exam – microscopic examination of tissue from a biopsy

Image Analysis and Computer-Assisted Diagnosis – Computer programs that can document and analyze the clinical and dermoscopic features of digitized pigmented lesion images, aiding in diagnosis.

Immunocytochemistry or immunohistochemistry (IHC) stains – Special stains that can highlight melanoma cells, refining Mohs surgeons' ability to identify them. These stains use substances such as frozen tissue sections of melanoma antigen recognized by T cells (MART-1), which preferentially stick to pigment cells (melanocytes) where melanoma occurs, making them much easier to see with the microscope.

Immunotherapy (biologic therapy or biotherapy) – The use of drugs that act on or involve the body's immune system in battling advanced cancers.

In situ – Latin words meaning "in place," used to describe the earliest melanomas that are limited to the uppermost part of the epidermis and have not invaded below the skin surface.

Interferons (IFNs) – A class of proteins produced by the immune system to stop the growth of viruses, tumors, and other foreign agents. Injectable interferon alfa-2b, a mass-produced lab version of IFN, was the first of two drugs with FDA approval for treating "high-risk" Stage II and Stage III melanomas.

Interleukin-2 (IL-2, also called Proleukin® or aldesleukin) – A large protein molecule produced by white blood cells formed in the immune system. It is a lymphokine that activates other cells in the immune system. High-dose IL-2, a mass-produced lab version of IL-2, was the first (and until 2011 the only) FDA-approved immunotherapy used to treat Stage IV metastatic melanoma.

In-transit (or satellite) metastases – Melanoma that has spread more than two centimeters from the primary tumor, but has not reached the nearby lymph nodes.

Invasive tumor – A tumor that penetrates into the deeper skin structures, the lymph nodes, or the internal organs.

Ipilimumab (Yervoy®) – *see* **Anti-CTLA-4 Therapy.**

Isolated Limb Perfusion – A treatment that relieves symptoms when melanoma metastases have reached an arm or leg. A chemotherapy drug, usually melphalan, is perfused (shunted directly) to the blood flowing through the affected limb, but to no other part of the body, to limit toxic effects.

Isosulfan blue – a blue dye used in lymph node mapping prior to sentinel node biopsy. The dye is injected into the skin around the tumor, and the dye passes into the lymph fluid, tracing its path. The blue color is picked up first by the node closest to the tumor, which is referred to as the sentinel node.

Keratin – A protein that is the principal component of skin, hair, and nails, providing structural support.

Keratinocytes – Epidermal cells that produce keratin.

Keratosis – A type of skin lesion in which there is overgrowth of horny tissue on the skin, as in actinic keratosis.

Lentigo – A benign flat brown spot occurring on the skin, often referred to inaccurately as a "liver spot." Found in about 80 percent of elderly people and in younger people who have had excessive sun exposure.

Lentigo maligna – A type of melanoma in situ that grows horizontally on the surface of sun-exposed areas, usually the face of elderly people. One of the four basic types of melanoma.

Lentigo maligna melanoma – The invasive form of lentigo maligna.

Lesion – A skin abnormality, such as a regular mole, atypical mole, precancer, or skin cancer, which is sometimes congenital but more often caused by an injury or sun exposure. Usually, it is first restricted to a specific area of the skin, but if not treated, cancerous lesions can spread, or metastasize, to other parts of the body.

Ligand – a molecule that binds to another (usually larger) receptor molecule.

Longitudinal melanonychia – a dark brown-to-black streak that extends from the cuticle to the tip of the nail, it is often a sign of nail bed melanoma.

Lymph nodes – Bean-shaped or round structures found along the course of the lymph channels, where lymph is filtered and lymphocytes are formed. The lymph vessels drain into the channels.

Lymphocytes – Small leukocytes (white blood cells) formed in lymphatic tissue with a single round nucleus.

Lymphokines – Substances released by lymphocytes in response to stimulation by an antigen. Part of the immune system.

Lymphoscintigraphy – A technique for mapping the lymphatic pathway to help track whether melanoma cells have metastasized from the primary tumor to the local lymph nodes. A radioactive substance, often along with a blue dye, is injected at the primary site, and a scanner traces the flow of lymph fluid draining from it to the nodes.

Lymphoseek (technetium Tc99m tilmanocept) – the first new radioactive tracer for lymph node mapping to be FDA-approved in more than 30 years, it is especially effective at locating the lymph nodes.

Lymph vessels – Vessels containing a clear liquid that bathes body cells. It contains white blood cells (lymphocytes) and a few red blood cells.

Malignant – Cancerous.

MC1R (melanocortin 1 receptor) gene – Popularly known as the red-headed gene. Variants in this gene are associated with an increased risk of both melanoma and basal cell carcinoma.

MDM2 – a recently discovered gene which, when mutated and in the presence of estrogen, may increase a woman's propensity for developing melanoma, especially at younger ages.

MelaFind®— A non-invasive, objective computer vision system FDA-approved in 2011, it is intended to aid in early detection of melanoma. It acquires and displays multi-spectral digital images of pigmented skin lesions and employs automated image analysis and statistical pattern recognition to help identify lesions and diagnose or rule out melanoma.

Melanin – Pigment that gives color to the skin, hair, and eyes. When the skin is damaged by the sun, it produces more melanin, evidenced by a tan. Scientists now know that there are two distinctly different types of melanin. Most people have *eumelanin* ("good" melanin), associated with the black/brown pigments found in people with skin that does not burn as easily and is not as vulnerable to skin cancer. Some, however, such as Celtic people with red hair and very light skin that cannot tan, have *pheomelanin,* which is associated with red/yellow pigments and is much more vulnerable to rapid sunburn, skin damage, and skin cancer.

Melanocytes – The melanin-producing cells in the basal layer of the epidermis.

Melanoma – The most serious form of skin cancer, originating in melanocytes that have become malignant. Also known as "malignant melanoma" or "cutaneous melanoma."

Metastasis – Spread of cancer cells from one part of the body to another, usually via the blood or lymph vessels.

Microarray technologies – techniques that allow scientists to screen large numbers of genes, closely examining DNA on the molecular level. Researchers seek to harness these technologies to measure and catalog patterns of gene mutation in different lesions, to help distinguish melanomas from benign moles or other cancers.

Micrometastases— Metastases so tiny that they can be seen only through the microscope.

Mitotic rate – The speed of cell division in a tumor, essentially how fast the tumor is growing. In the new American Joint Committee on Cancer (AJCC) melanoma staging system, the presence of at least one mitosis (cancer cell division) per millimeter squared (mm^2) can upgrade a thin melanoma to a later stage.

Mohs micrographic surgery – A surgical method of excising skin cancer in which each layer of tissue removed is studied under the microscope during surgery for the presence of cancer cells. When the last layer removed is cancer-free, the surgery ends. Mohs has been shown to be the single most effective technique for certain nonmelanoma skin cancers, and can also be used with certain melanomas.

Moles – Pigmented lesions on the skin. Normal moles are benign growths of melanocytes. Also called "nevi."

Monoclonal antibody – This type of antibody binds or attaches itself to one specific antigen. For this reason, it is often mass-produced in laboratories for use in diagnosis and treatment.

Mortality rate – The number of deaths per year per 100,000 population that can b attributed to a specific cause.

MRI (Magnetic resonance imaging) scan – An imaging technique that uses a mag net instead of an X ray to create a map of the patient's body and brain.

MSLT-1 and MSLT-2 (the Multicenter Selective Lymphadenectomy Trial–and Trial-2) – Two long-running studies of sentinel lymph node biopsy research ing whether it improves survival statistics for melanoma patients in whom metas tases have reached the lymph nodes. The results of MSLT-1 did not prove extende overall survival or melanoma-specific survival, but did show that SLNB is associated with improved *recurrence*-free survival (the length of time before recurrence) The results of MSLT-2 are not yet in.

Nail (subungual) melanoma – a type of acral lentiginous melanoma that typically shows up on the nails of the thumb or big toe either as a dark brown-to-black streal that extends from the cuticle to the tip of the nail (called *longitudinal melano nychia*), or as a so-called "colorless" tumor (known as *amelanotic melanoma)* tha may actually be red, pink, purple, or normal skin tone. Nail melanomas are ofter mistaken for less serious conditions until advanced, leading to poorer outcomes.

Nevus – A pigmented or unpigmented common mole on the skin. The plural i "nevi."

Nivolumab (Opdivo®) – *see* **anti-PD-1 therapy.**

Nodular melanoma – One of the four basic types of melanoma, accounting for 1 to 15 percent of all melanomas. Usually invasive when diagnosed, it is the mos aggressive of the melanomas. It most frequently occurs on the trunk, legs, an arms, especially in elderly people.

Nodule – A rounded growth that protrudes above the surface of the skin.

Nonmalignant – Benign, not cancerous.

Nonmelanoma – The overall name for skin cancers other than melanomas. The mos common forms are basal cell carcinomas and squamous cell carcinomas.

Oncogenes – Cancer-producing genes.

Oncologist – A physician who specializes in the diagnosis and especially the treat ment of cancers or tumors.

Organs – Important body structures, internal and external — for example, the skin, eyes, liver, and kidneys.

Ozone – A gas made up of three oxygen atoms. It forms a layer in the stratosphere that keeps some ultraviolet rays (including virtually all UVC rays) from reaching the earth's surface.

Palpable nodes – lymph nodes that the physician can feel on physical examination. These swollen nodes may indicate that a melanoma has reached the lymph nodes.

Papillary dermis – The upper portion of the second layer of skin, directly below the epidermis.

Papule – A small bump on the skin. Skin cancers may initially appear as papules.

Pathology – The laboratory study of cells and tissues to determine and diagnose disease.

PD-1– *see* **anti-PD-1 therapy.**

PD-L1 (programmed death ligand-1) – One of two ligands for the protein receptor PD-1. When PD-L1 binds to PD-1, it prevents T cells from attacking melanoma and other cancers. The new anti-PD-1 therapies can prevent these ligands from binding to PD-1, thereby allowing T cells to attack the cancer: see anti-PD-1 therapy. Anti-PD-L1 therapies specifically targeting PD-L1 are now also being researched; one such experimental therapy, an engineered antibody called MPDL3280A, can prevent PD-L1 from binding to PD-1, thereby allowing T cells to be released.

Pegylated interferon alfa-2b (peginterferon alfa-2b, or Sylatron™) – an improved, recently FDA-approved version of IFN alfa-2b for Stage II and Stage III high-risk melanoma patients. Injected subcutaneously, this enhanced version of IFN alfa-2b has longer-lasting effects than the original form, enabling patients to remain relapse-free longer.

Pembrolizumab (Keytruda®) – *see* **anti-PD-1 therapy.**

PET (positron emission tomography) scan – A powerful diagnostic tool that detects melanoma cells by showing whether they take up radioactive sugar.

Photosensitivity – Increased sensitivity of the skin to sunlight and other sources of UV.

Primary tumor – A first-time malignancy that has not been treated.

Prognosis – A forecast of the probable outcome of a disease — cure, improvement, remission, or continuation, advance, recurrence, or death.

Radiation therapy – Use of X rays to destroy malignant and benign growths. In melanoma patients, radiation therapy is usually reserved for patients who are not good candidates for surgery due to age or other health concerns.

Radical node dissection – removal of all lymph nodes in a lymph node basin.

Reconstruction – The repair of defects on the skin after the removal of a lesion.

Resect – To cut or remove a tumor or other structures such as lymph nodes.

Resistance – The adaptive ability of malignant cells to withstand the effects o. toxic agents targeted against them.

Reticular dermis – The lower portion of the second layer of skin.

Sentinel node (sentinel lymph node) – The lymph node nearest to a primary mela noma, it is the first place where metastasis is likely to occur.

Sentinel lymph node biopsy (SLNB) – A biopsy of the node(s) nearest to a primary tumor, to determine whether cancer cells have metastasized beyond the primary site. Such a biopsy is now frequently done when a tumor is more than 1 mm i thickness, shows evidence of ulceration, or has a mitotic rate of at least one mitosi (cancer cell division) per millimeter squared (mm^2).

SIMSYS-MoleMate™ SIAscope™ (Spectrophotometric Intracutaneou: Analysis System) – A handheld device that uses both visible and infrared light t examine skin components such as blood, melanin, and collagen to a depth of 2 mn below the skin surface, providing living pathological data on skin lesions. Using so phisticated mathematical models and software programs, it generates images called SIAscans, which demonstrate how skin features relate to one another. This allow physicians to know the exact size of a lesion and make more precise incisions.

Solar radiation – Light rays, both visible and invisible, produced by the sun.

SPF (sun protection factor) – a measurement of how well a sunscreen protect: against the sun's ultraviolet B rays and sunburn. Optimally, individuals using sun screen with an SPF of 15 can go 15 times longer in the sun without burning fron UVB than they would without the sunscreen.

Squamous cell carcinoma – A skin cancer made up of cells resembling those foun in the mid-portion of the epidermis. The second most common form of skin cancer

Staging – Dividing patients into groups (stages), based on the severity and stag of advance of their disease, from Stage I to Stage IV. Melanoma classification wa: developed by the American Joint Commission on Cancer (AJCC).

Stratum corneum – The rough or scaly (horny) outermost layer of the epidermis consisting of flat dead or peeling cells.

Subungual melanoma – *see* **nail melanoma.**

Superficial spreading melanoma – The most common type of melanoma, whicl appears on the surface of the skin as an irregularly shaped, colored or changing growing mole.

Understanding Melanom.

Surgical margins – The surrounding, presumably cancer-free borders of the entire area where a tumor has been excised. Today, the margins tend to be much narrower than in the past, meaning that much less tissue is removed, presumably with no added risk of metastasis. However, some scientists are now questioning whether margins have become *too* narrow.

Survival rate – The percentage of people who are alive at a certain time after melanoma diagnosis, for example, after one, five, and ten years.

Talimogene laherparepvec (T-VEC) – a form of oncolytic virus (a modified herpes virus that cannot infect the patient) injected directly into tumors to preferentially infect the cancer cells, rupturing their cell walls while leaving healthy cells intact. The hope is that as the tumor disintegrates, it will release infectious virus particles, stimulating inflammatory signals that broadly activate the immune system to attack other, non-inoculated tumors. A 2014 Phase III study produced a 16 percent response rate vs. 2 percent in untreated control patients.

Targeted therapy – A therapy meant to attack or alter a specific, biologically important process, gene, or molecule that is believed to play a part in a disease. Such therapies often have better results and produce fewer side effects than general systemic chemotherapy, which attacks healthy cells along with diseased cells.

T cells – Lymphocytes produced by the thymus that are particularly important to the immune response.

Trametinib (Mekinist™) – an FDA-approved oral targeted inhibitor of MEK 1 and 2 (mitogen-activated protein kinase kinase 1 and 2) indicated as a single agent and in combination with the BRAF inhibitor dabrafenib, for the treatment of patients with inoperable or metastatic melanoma with BRAF V600E or V600K mutations. By specifically binding to MEK, trametinib inhibits cell signaling and cellular proliferation in melanoma. Patients on combined dabrafenib and trametinib have been found to have significantly prolonged progression-free survival compared to those on dabrafenib alone.

Tumor – A swelling or overgrowth of tissue. May be cancerous or benign.

Tumor-infiltrating lymphocytes (TILs) – TILs are immune cells that act in response to a tumor. In one form of immunotherapy, they can be removed from a patient's tumor, grown and multiplied in the lab, then reinjected in quantity into the patient to help fight a cancer. In some studies, genetic material is added to the TILs to produce growth factors that make the TILs more aggressive before being returned to the patient's body.

Ugly Duckling Sign – A new method for visual detection of skin lesions that could be melanomas. It is based on the concept that melanomas are "ugly ducklings" or outliers that look or feel different, or evolve differently than surrounding moles.

Ulceration – The epidermis above a large part of the melanoma is not intact. When a melanoma is ulcerated, it can upgrade the tumor to a more advanced stage.

Ultraviolet (UV) rays – Invisible light waves radiating from the sun or an artificial source, such as a sunlamp or tanning bed. UVA, UVB, and UVC are the three types of UV rays, but only UVA and UVB reach the earth. About 90 percent of all skin cancers and premature skin aging are attributable to the sun's UVA and UVB rays.

UPF – Ultraviolet Protection Factor, a special rating for clothing, similar to SPF. UPF indicates how much of the sun's UV radiation is absorbed. A fabric with a rating of 50 will allow only 1/50th of the sun's UV rays to pass through.

UVA – The longest ultraviolet rays, having a wavelength of 320–400 nanometers. (A nanometer equals one-billionth of a meter.) Equally damaging year-round, UVA rays penetrate into the skin deeper than UVB, and have been strongly linked to premature aging, as well as to melanoma and other skin cancers.

UVB – The shorter ultraviolet rays, having a wavelength of 290–320 nanometers. UVB is the wavelength primarily responsible for sunburn, and along with UVA rays, plays a part in photoaging, skin cancers, eye damage, and immune system suppression.

UV Index – An estimate of the peak amount of ultraviolet radiation reaching the earth's surface at solar noon. The higher the UV Index on a given day, the more intense the sun's UV rays reaching earth that day.

Vaccine – Unlike the vaccines given to prevent disease, melanoma vaccines are a treatment for patients who have the disease. They stimulate the immune system to fight off the cancer. Many are still being tested.

Vemurafenib (Zelboraf®) – a targeted drug inhibitor of the defective BRAF gene, which occurs in about half of melanoma patients. In patients with the defective BRAF gene, vemurafenib can bind to the defective protein and deactivate it. It can produce rapid, striking antitumor activity in patients with BRAF V600E- and V600K-mutated melanoma, leading to both a progression-free and overall survival (OS) advantage compared to patients on standard chemotherapy. However, most patients eventually develop resistance to the treatment, and the melanoma starts to advance again.

VivaScope 3000 – a form of confocal scanning laser microscopy that employs miniaturized, user-friendly handheld scanners. See confocal scanning laser microscopy.

PHOTOGRAPHS AND ILLUSTRATIONS

The ABCDEs of Moles and Melanomas, The Skin Cancer Foundation, ©2006, revised 2014

American Cancer Society, Surveillance and Health Policy Research, 2009. http://www.cancer.org/acs/groups/content/@nho/documents/document/cff2009probdevcancer7pdf.pdf

Basal Cell Carcinoma, The Skin Cancer Foundation, 1986, revised 1999, 2003, 2007, 2014

David G. Brodland, MD

William A. Crutcher, MD

Mona Gohara, MD

If You Can Spot It, You Can Stop It, The Skin Cancer Foundation, ©1992, revised 2011

The Many Faces of Melanoma, The Skin Cancer Foundation, 1985, revised 1996, 2010

Lifetime Risk of Invasive Melanoma, Graph. Rigel DS, et al, NYU Melanoma Cooperative Group

Maritza Perez, MD

Squamous Cell Carcinoma, The Skin Cancer Foundation, 1990, revised 1999, 2003, 2008, 2010, 2014

Cross-section of Skin. *Sun Sense,* Perry Robins, MD
The Skin Cancer Foundation, ©1990, page 17

The 2006 *Skin Cancer Foundation Journal.* ©2006, Page 20.
Reprinted with permission Ashfaq A. Marghoob, MD

The 2013 *Skin Cancer Foundation Journal.* ©2013, Page 63.
Reprinted with permission Ashfaq A. Marghoob, MD

The 2014 *Skin Cancer Foundation Journal.* ©2014, Page 32.
Reprinted with permission Maral K. Skelsey, MD

Anatomical Distribution, NYU Melanoma Cooperative Group
The 1986 *Skin Cancer Foundation Journal*, page 25

Momtaz P, Lacouture ME, Chapman PB. Current Choices and Strategies in the Treatment of Metastatic Melanoma. *The Melanoma Letter,* spring 2014, Vol. 32, page 2.

INDEX

Environmental Protection Agency, 64

Epidermis 3, 5, 10, 11-12, 13

Epiluminescence microscopy 8, *also see* Dermoscopy

Estrogen 43, 70

Eumelanin 43-44

Excision, *see* Surgery

Exercise 16, 60

Family 41-45, 59, 61, 66

Family Syndrome 42

Family, melanoma-prone 29, 41-45, 46-47, 68-69

Fascia 17

Food and Drug Administration (FDA) 9-10, 15, 20, 22-28, 52, 67-68

Gender 54-57

Gene mutations 8, 27-28, 42-44, 49, 58

Gene therapy 28-30, 68-69

Genome (melanoma) 8, 49

Grafts 16

Hawaii 5, 50, 56, 66

Helping Hand newsletter 61

Heredity 41, 66

Hispanics 56

Histologic examination 8

Hormones 44, 47, 69, 70

Image analysis 9-10

Imatinib 28, 30

Immunotherapy 20, 22, 23-30, 67-68

In situ melanomas 3, 4-5, 12-13, 16

Incidence 4, 5, 44, 48, 50, 54-57

Interferon alfa-2b 23, 64, 67

Interleukin-2 23, 24, 67

Intermediate melanomas 12, 13

Internal organs 13-14, 21, 66

International Agency for Research on Cancer 51

Internet 59-60, 64, *also see* Support groups

In-transit metastasis 13-14, 21

Invasive melanomas 3, 4-6, 44, 54-55

Ipilimumab 24-27, 29-30, 67-68

Isolated limb perfusion 22-23

Keytruda, see Pembrolizumab

Laboratory studies 7-8, 19, 20, 29, 65

Lentigo maligna 5, 6, 50

Lesions 7-10, 32, 33, 55, 57, 58, 65

Lymph node, sentinel, *see* sentinel node

Lymph nodes 12, 13-14, 18-23, 66-67, 69, 70

Lymph 13, 19, 20, 66

Lymphocytes 24, 29, 68

Lymphodepletion 24

Lymphokine 23

Lymphoscintigraphy 19-20

MAPK pathway 27-28, 42-43

Margins, surgical 15, 16-18

MART-1 17

MC1R 29, 43-44, 68

MDM2 43

MEK 27-28, 43, 68

Mekinist, *see* Trametinib

MelaFind® 10

Melanin 3, 10, 43-44, 52, 55

Melanocortin 1 receptor (MC1R) gene 29, 43-44, 68

Melanocytes 3, 17-18, 65, 70

Melphalan 23

Membership, Skin Cancer Foundation 71

Metastasis 11, 13-14, 17, 19, 21, 22, 24, 26, 28, 29, 66-68, 70

Microarray technologies 8

Micrometastases 14

Mitotic rate 11-13, 19, 66

Mohs micrographic surgery 17-18

Moles 1, 3, 4, 7-8, 31-34, 37, 41-45, 49, 65, 66, 69, 70, *also see* Atypical moles

Monoclonal antibody 24-5, 67

Mortality rate 55, *also see* Survival rate

MRI 21, 67

Multicenter Selective Lymphadenectomy Trial (MSLT) 20-21

Multi-spectral imaging 10

Mutations, *see* Gene mutations

Nail melanoma 5-6, 9, 32-33, 56

Narrow excision 16-17

National Cancer Institute 24, 47

National Institutes of Health 16

National Oceanic and Atmospheric Administration 64

Nevi, *see* Moles

Nilotinib 28, 30

Nivolumab 25-6, 29, 68

Nodular melanoma 6, 32, 33

Nonmelanomas, *see* Basal cell carcinomas, Squamous cell carcinomas

Nutrition, *see* Diet

Oncolytic viruses 27

Opdivo, *see* Nivolumab

Palpation 14, 18-19, 66

Papillary dermis 10

Pathologist 5, 7

Pathology laboratory 7, 19, 20

PD-1 25-6, 68

Peginterferon 23, 67

Pembrolizumab 25-6, 29, 30, 68

PET scan 21, 67

Pheomelanin 44

Pigment 3, 5, 8-10, 17, 32, 33, 43-44, 55, 65

Pigmented lesions 8-10, 33

Pregnancy 44, 46, 69, 70

Prevention 22, 26, 37, 43, 56, 62-64

Primary 13-14, 15, 16, 18, 19, 21, 66, 69, 70

Programmed death-1, *see* PD-1

Prognosis 5, 11, 20, 55, *also see* Survival rate

Proleukin 23, *also see* Interleukin-2

Puberty 44, 45, 46

Radial growth phase 5

Radical node dissection 19-21

Recurrence 21, 27, 59, 60, 67, 69, 70

Redheads, *see* Pheomelanin

Resection, *see* Surgery

Resistance 27, 28

Risk factors 41-46, 48-53, 54, 56, 57, 62, 64, 66, *also see* Family

Risk, lifetime 54-55

Satellite metastasis, *see* In-transit metastasis

Scars 7, 15-16

Self-examination 31-40, 44-47, 56, 63, 65, 66

Sentinel node biopsy (SLNB) 13, 16, 19-21, 66, 70

Sentinel node, 13, 16, 19-21, 66-67, 70

Sex 60

SIAscope™ 10

Skin Cancer Foundation, 35, 56, 62, 63, 64, 70 71, 72

SkinCancer.org 71

Skin color 6, 43-44, 50-51, 52-53, 55, 56, 64, 66

Skin self-examination, *see* Self-examination

Skin types 52-53, 56

Squamous cell carcinomas 2, 17, 35, 37, 48, 51, 55, 70

Squamous cells 3

Stages 11-14, 20-23

Stains 5, 8, 17-18

Subungual melanoma, *see* Nail melanoma

Sun exposure 6, 46, 49-52, 66, 70-71

Sun protection 46, 47, 50, 62-64. 70-71

Sun Protection Factor (SPF) 47, 58, 63, 71

Sunburn 42, 44, 49-51, 56, 63, 66